I0001173

Richard Barwell

The causes and treatment of lateral curvature of the spine

Richard Barwell

The causes and treatment of lateral curvature of the spine

ISBN/EAN: 9783742826930

Manufactured in Europe, USA, Canada, Australia, Japa

Cover: Foto ©Lupo / pixelio.de

Manufactured and distributed by brebook publishing software
(www.brebook.com)

Richard Barwell

The causes and treatment of lateral curvature of the spine

THE
CAUSES AND TREATMENT
OF
LATERAL CURVATURE OF THE SPINE.

By RICHARD BARWELL, F.R.C.S.,

SURGEON TO AND LECTURER ON ANATOMY AT THE CHARING CROSS HOSPITAL.

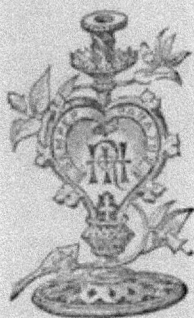

ENLARGED FROM LECTURES PUBLISHED IN 'THE LANCET.'

LONDON:

ROBERT HARDWICKE, 192, PICCADILLY.

1868.

PREFACE.

ALTHOUGH it be unadvisable that an author should in a preface argue the necessity of reading his book, he may nevertheless be permitted to state why it has been written. In the present plethora of medical literature no one should publish unless he has something to say which he believes to be more than a mere repetition of what has been said in another form,—something which he believes to be both new and useful. The reason of my having such faith in the ensuing pages may be thus stated.

Having failed to find in books a satisfactory theory of those conditions which produce lateral curvature, it naturally appeared that in all the works, English and continental, which I studied, and whose name is legion, there was something defective, for they gave, to my thinking, no explanation of certain

essential peculiarities of that deformity. Endeavouring to carry further their line of
reasoning, the same gap or the same impas-
sable barrier presented itself. It then appeared
that, to carry out my desire, I must work for
myself. To do this I first examined a great
many normal backs under different conditions,
measuring and calculating different movements
and varying postures, both at rest and in
exercise. The results of about twenty months
of this labour are given in a few lines of the
ensuing pages; at the same time, dissections
and examinations of normal and morbid specimens, as far as my opportunities would permit,
were carried on. Having completed these
studies, I turned to living spinal curvatures,
and investigated their condition with the insight which my studies of the norm had
afforded. This work also occupied a considerable period, during which time all theorizing
was avoided until a large mass of facts were
collected, until these facts presented me with
a causation which I could trust, and until
experience led me to a treatment calculated to
remedy its effects. Although, then, a great

deal has been written upon the subject of lateral curvature of the spine, I yet hold myself justified in adding another work to the list; because the views which I have been led to form account for those essential characteristics which have been hitherto left unexplained, and because the treatment which I advocate is certainly less irksome, and will, I firmly believe, be found by others, as by myself, more efficacious than that which has hitherto been pursued.

It only remains for me to say that the substance, or, as it may be called, a summary, of the ensuing pages, appeared in 'The Lancet' during the latter end of the last and the beginning of the present year. Perhaps may be partly due to that form of publication a certain mode of arrangement which, though not quite logical or orderly, will, I think, conduce to the more easy comprehension of the doctrine which I desire to teach.

RICHARD BARWELL.

32, *George Street, Hanover Square,*
    26th May, 1868.

CONTENTS.

CHAPTER I.

THE NORMAL SPINE.

Characteristics of Curvature — Theories of **Curvature** — Formation of spine — Erect attitude — Cause **of normal curves** — Measurement of **normal** curves — Form of **vertebræ** — Action of ligaments — Rotatory power of the spine — Lateral flexibility — Influence of limb-motion — Axis of rotation — Conditions of deformity curable and incurable .. **Page 1**

CHAPTER II.

CAUSES OF DORSAL CURVATURE.

Definitions — At present unexplained — Rotatory acts — Action of Serratus — Respiratory and weight-bearing — Lever-like action of ribs — Torsion the first step — Influence of dress — Influence of stays — The secondary curves   **26**

CHAPTER III.

CAUSES OF LUMBAR CURVATURE.

Undulatory movements of spine — Obliquity of pelvis — Distribution of weight — Uneven tension of thighs — Action of lumbar muscles — Effects of Myotomy **48**

CHAPTER IV.

DIAGNOSIS OF DIFFERENT CURVES.

Prominence of hip — Of shoulder — Presence of any curve — Direction of light — Differential diagnosis — Dorsal — Lumbar — Rotation — Lateral deviation — Anterior changes in form — Uneven rotation power — Diagnosis between weight-bearing and respiratory curve — Position as cause of curve —Earliest signs of curvatures   ..   Page 59

CHAPTER V.

SIGNS OF CURABILITY.

Significance of muscular changes — Changes in spine are secondary — Measurements of vertebræ, &c., in distortion — Elasticity of ligaments, &c. — Effects of Recumbency   81

CHAPTER VI.

PRINCIPLES OF TREATMENT.

Prevalent treatment — Its misdirection — The spinal support —Construction and defects — Opinion of its fautors — New method — Its rationale — Direction of force in supports — Variable postures — Remedial positions   90

CHAPTER VII.

TREATMENT OF LUMBAR CURVATURE.

Proportioned to amount of curve — Sloping seat — Its effects — High-shoe — Exercises — Lumbar bandage —Regulation of treatment — Cases   106

CHAPTER VIII.

TREATMENT OF DORSAL CURVATURE.

Weight-bearing curves — Divisions of treatment — The shoulder-sling — Remedial postures — Exercises — Difference in cases — Respiratory curve — Arrangement of dress — Positions — Sloping seat — Lateral sling — Exercises — Abdominal movements — Respiratory exercise — Swing of arm — Oblique bandage — Regulation of treatment — Medicinal interference — Cases — Estimates by rotation — Measure — By perpendicular line .. .. Page 129

CHAPTER IX.

SEVERE AND SLIGHT CURVATURE.

Exaggerated curve — From usual causes — From internal cause — Example from early lung-disease — Pains in exaggerated curve — The spiral bandage — Examples of its value — Slight curve — Non-symptomatic postures of scapula — Hysteric spine 159

INDEX 173

ON LATERAL CURVATURE
OF THE SPINE.

CHAPTER I.

THE NORMAL SPINE.

THE treatises which I have published on
Diseases of Joints, and on Clubfoot, &c., will
probably lead those of my readers who are
acquainted with their contents, to expect in
the ensuing pages a somewhat analogous
mode of dealing with deformities of the trunk.
This, I believe, will be found to be the case,
not only in my endeavours to assign the malady
to its real cause, but also in the *direct* method
of treatment advocated. It may be permitted
me to recall the fact, that in my writings on
the subjects first named I have insisted on
the necessity of going beyond the mere forcing
of immobile parts into a position, which they
must either retain, with permanent immobility
or abrogate with resumption of motion—that

B

I have especially advocated treatment during
the continuance of functional movement in
such manner as to prevent destruction of joint
structures, more especially the fatty fibrous
degeneration of muscle so certain to attack
those organs while retained in forced repose—
and that in doing this it has been my task
to point out some muscular functions and
actions hitherto overlooked or insufficiently
considered; but upon which the persistence
of the malady nevertheless depends.

Cotemporarily with my investigations on
joints and limbs, I began to study English
and Continental works on the spine; and
soon became involved in a haze of diffi-
culties and a fog of contradictions—since of
all the irreconcileable theories on the causes
of lateral curvature, not a single one of them,
nor all put together, account for the peculiarities of the disease.* These peculiarities
are so constant and so remarkable as to in-

---

* Of course we must here except the curvature of
rachitic origin, and those resulting from internal in-
flammations. I am speaking only of lateral curvature
as a primary disease.

spire a true and instinctive feeling, that if they be left unexplained the disease itself is not understood. At the risk of forestalling points that must be examined hereafter, it will be necessary to mention the three most important characteristics of lateral curvature, and to contrast them with the explanations hitherto given. These are torsion of vertebræ,* predominance of dorsal curvature to one and the same side, and tendency to affect chiefly almost exclusively the female sex, and among these hardly any but women of Europe and the United States — especially of the Northern States. It would make this work utterly unreadable to mention all the theories that have been formed to account for these conditions; but it may be possible to do them full justice, without boring the reader, by classifying them into spastic contraction, debility and paralysis of spinal muscles, paralysis of respi-

---

* That is to say, each aberrant vertebra is twisted horizontally, so that the anterior surface of its body looks to the convexity, the tips of its spinous processes to the concavity of the curve. The degree of curvature corresponding accurately with the amount of torsion.

ratory muscles, overaction of the right arm,
uneven distribution of the weight of the trunk,
the weight of the heart hanging on the dorsal,
that of the liver on the lumbar spine—disease
and deformation of vertebræ and of intervertebral substance.* Now the difficulty with
all these is as follows :—they none of them
account, or indeed attempt to account, for rotation. If any one of these theories, except the
over-action of right arm or weighting by heart
and liver, were correct, the dorsal curvature
must of necessity be as frequently to the left
as to the right. The theory of over-use of
the right arm, even were it for a moment
tenable, should make the affection more usual
in men than in women. The different weighting of the column by liver and heart should,
if it were the efficient cause, render lateral
curvature a constant and usual condition,
equally common in both sexes. Thus, as we
examine each and every of these theories, we

---

* I believe every theory will be found to range
itself within one or the other of these classes—over-
weight of head being accepted as equal to debility,
—Lack of nutrition as equivalent to disease.

find one or more of the characteristics in
the disease unexplained; and as these points
are not accidents, but essentials, the disease as
a whole is not elucidated.

I believe that, in the course of the ensuing
pages, I shall be able to give a satisfactory
explanation of this perplexed subject, and to
show how, upon a correct pathology, a more
efficacious and less irksome or injurious treatment is to be adopted than the present prevalent method of screwing the spine into iron
splints. To do this fairly we must take up
the subject from early physiology, since by
that means alone can we determine what
forces act, and how they act on the vertebral
column.

The bodies of the twenty-four bones com-
posing the spine are placed alternately with
intervertebral ligaments, so as to form a continuous column, which, lying within the
abdomen, within the chest, and behind the
gullet, tapers with slight modifications from
below upwards to the point upon which the
head is pivoted. The vertebræ, separated
from each other in front by the remarkably

elastic intervertebral ligament, only touch at
the back of the spinal canal by the small facets
on the articular processes, one on each side.
Each bone, therefore, rests upon its fellow by
a tripod, between the feet of which lies the
axis of motion, and where the vertebral
canal perforates the bone. Movement at the
articular surfaces takes place by the gliding
action common to these and all arthrodial
joints; the movement between the bodies is
produced by compression, stretching, or twisting of the intervertebral substance which is
thick enough to suffer these alterations to
a very great extent, and elastic enough to
recover them completely.

Now the spine of the infant is intrinsically
straight in all directions; while so very young
as to be kept always recumbent, the back,
perfectly devoid of any inherent bend, merely
follows the curves of the surface upon which
the child lies. The pelvis is nearly horizontal,
i. e. the brim of the true pelvis projects at
little more than a right angle from the lumbar
spine. When the infant sits up on the nurse's
arm the back bends in one single antero-

posterior curve, concavity to the front, the
pelvis maintaining the same relative position.

When, however, the child begins to walk,
a change takes place in all these postures.
The thighs must take a new position, and lie in
a line parallel with the body's axis. In doing
this they drag on all the muscles passing from
the anterior part of the os innominatum to the
femur—on the iliacus, rectus, pectineus, and
others; the pelvis, yielding to these forces,
must necessarily receive a downward slope,
and the sacrum must project backwards. The
psoas, made tense by the same force, draws
the loins forward, while the mass of lumbar
muscles enforces that bend of the lumbar
region necessary to compensate for the pelvic
obliquity, and to preserve the body in equi-
librio. It seems at first sight well to say that
the dorsal bend is produced by the necessity
of balance; but it will, on consideration, be
seen that there must be muscular force to place
the passive bones in the position which permits balance. This force is supplied by the
abdominal muscles, which passing from the
pelvis to the walls of the chest, are rendered

tense by the new posture of the former and descent of the pubic bones above described. On the front of the dorsal spine are no muscles,—for if any were so placed, their action through the vertebræ upon such long levers as the ribs would destroy that regularity of movement necessary for healthy breathing. Therefore each pair of ribs is not moved by muscles acting on the fore part of the spine : on the contrary, nearly all motion of that portion of the column is confided to muscles attached to the ribs.

The flexion backward of the cervical spine, also necessary for balance, is produced by the tension, employed for keeping the head erect, of those muscles which are attached to the occiput, as well as of those attached to the vertebræ themselves. I must here make an observation on the position of the head in man, and the small size of the ligamentum nuchæ, which is especially placed in animals to economise muscular power. Although the weight of the head is in man considerably forward, yet very little muscular power is required to keep it upright. The disposition of the upper part of the trapezius muscle, running from occiput to acromion, is such that a small part of the weight of the shoulders is quite sufficient to counterbalance the forward tendency of the head; the muscle is not fatigued thereby, since no contraction, further than mere tonic tension, is necessary to permit the weight of the one part to act on the gravity of the other.

When the adult or adolescent stands erect, with the weight evenly distributed between the two feet, the antero-posterior curves of the spine are three—cervical, dorsal, and lumbar, which alternate in direction; they may be thus expressed :—

CERVICAL—convex in front, 28 degrees of a circle of $6\frac{5}{8}$ radius, begins at the odontoid process, and ends at middle of 2nd dorsal vertebræ.

DORSAL—convex behind, 42 degrees of a circle of $12\frac{2}{8}$ radius, begins at 2nd dorsal, ends lower edge of 11th dorsal.

LUMBAR—convex in front, 80 degrees of a circle of $5\frac{3}{8}$ radius, begins middle last dorsal, ends lower edge last lumbar.

The chords of these arcs lie in one continuous line, which is the perpendicular of the crooked column ; or to put it in other words, a perpendicular drawn from the tip of the odontoid process impinges on the vertebræ above-named, and forms the chords of the vertebral curves. This line, traced onwards beyond the lumbar vertebræ, falls at right angles on the centre of a line drawn from the middle of one acetabulum across the pelvis to the other. Thus the weight of the body falls upon the strong transverse arch formed by the thick ilio-pectineal line, and thence is transferred to another transverse arch, constructed by the necks of the thigh bones.

A considerable portion of the lateral springiness of the trunk is produced by these transverse arches : one buttress can be raised from the solid ground, and slung as it were upon resilient muscular power.

The above-mentioned incurvation of the spine has generally been considered and described as an essential characteristic of the column ; but this is far from being the case ; it is simply a condition forced upon the bones by the human erect posture, and is essentially one of effort. This is proved by the congenital form of the spine, which is straight, by the fact that in lying down to sleep—even in sitting at ease—these curves, especially the lumbar, and to a great extent the cervical, are obliterated, and the column assumes simply one curve (concavity in front) from the last lumbar to about the fourth cervical vertebra. I cannot but think that the brothers Weber were, in their estimates of the dimensions of vertebræ, misled by their ideas of what ought to be the case, rather than guided by accurate measurement. They assert that the bodies of vertebræ vary in such wise (to put the matter shortly), that they are in all cases thicker on the convex part of the curve. Herr Hirschfeld, of Prague, a most accurate observer, could find no such variation; nor have I, in my measurements of a great many spines, been able to discover such differences as the Berlin anatomists have described.*

* It appears to me that the great elaboration and abstruse appearance in calculation of arcs and sines have caused this learned work (' Die menschliche

Again, if the vertebræ did really vary thus in thickness, the spine would maintain those curves during recumbency, and the infantile column would be bent. Moreover, the spine when erect would lose that mechanism of exquisitely counterbalanced springs which I am about to describe.

When the recumbent or sitting individual, whose spine, either nearly straight or forming a slight long bend, rises to his feet, the column changes its form in the manner described, and certain connecting structures are compressed or stretched. Let us first take those connected only with the bodies of the vertebræ—viz., intervertebral substance, anterior and posterior ligament. Imagine first the bones and the interposed substance piled one above the other, forming a straight line, with the ligaments in front and behind equally tense. Now bend the column for-

---

Gehwerkzeuge') to be accepted with too little examination. I have, in another publication ('A Treatise on Diseases of the Joints'), shown that the great power which these authors attribute to a supposed articular vacuum is quite unfounded.

wards: the front of the intervertebral substance becomes compressed, the anterior ligament relaxed; while at the back the
intervertebral substance is thickened, and the
posterior ligament stretched : thus, in both
back and front aspects of the column, there is
attempt to restore the straight condition.
But, besides these, we must consider the parts
connected with the processes, which, especially those attached to the arches, are extremely elastic, and so arranged that they
constantly, by their retractile power, tend to
draw the back parts of each bone nearer together—*i. e.*, to make the spine concave poste-
riorly. Thus they are, at the loins and neck,
at ease in the erect posture; the posterior
muscles are there extremely strong : in the
back they are tense, and always endeavouring
to obliterate the dorsal curve, and in that part
the muscles behind the column are comparatively very weak. Let us consider these
conditions, first, in extremes : suppose the
individual stoop or bend the trunk forcibly
in any direction; there are always on the
convex side ligaments stretched, on the con-

cave substance compressed, both endeavouring
to restore the straight line. Next, suppose
the individual, seated as man usually sits,
with the lumbar curve obliterated, the dorsal
one nearly so; imagine him starting up, and
the spine assuming its curves—that is to say,
all these ligamentous aids to motion, all these
alternations of tenseness, are called into play;
the spine becomes a spring, or a series of
springs, which sets itself, or, rather, which set
each other, allowing the brain to ride as in a
well-hung carriage, and giving to the figure,
expectant or in motion, that lithe activity
which could never have been produced if the
bones were a series of wedges such as the
Webers describe.

Finding, then, that the normal antero-
posterior bends do not result from the form
of the bones, but are superinduced upon the
previously straight spine simply by muscular
force, I wished to determine, firstly, the
amount of influence such muscles exercise, or,
in other words, the degree of mobility, which
the spine, under ordinary circumstances, possesses; secondly, the particular muscles pro-

ducing the movements in question; thirdly, the mode in which the usual movements of the body or limbs affected the spinal column.

In order to determine the capability of rotation in persons unaccustomed to gymnastic performances, I contrived a means of attaching a light upright rod to the upper end of the sternum and chest in such-wise that it should be quite uninfluenced by any movement of the shoulders; but should only and accurately follow the movement of the sternum from side to side. The upper end of the rod was, by jointed attachments, placed in communication with a dial-index. The person to be examined is seated on a chair, the pelvis well fixed, and, for greater security, the knees grasp between them a wooden pillar or bulkhead, so that all twist of the pelvis is impossible. This instrument then will exactly indicate the amount of rotation of the loins and back, the neck not being included. A very general amount of this rotation is between 30° and 40° to either side. Occasionally one comes across persons who can only turn 25° each way, but it is more usual to meet with those whose power

exceeds 50°. I myself can turn 56°. One of
my subjects, seventeen years old, could turn
62° to each side — that is, more than one-
third of the circle.

If we assume that the power of rotation is
equally apportioned between the first dorsal
and fourth. lumbar vertebra (the last has no
power of rotation, in all probability), it would
be distributed amongst sixteen bones—that is,
each would revolve upon the other, 7° 75′.*

I tried also to measure the lateral curve
which the spine without absolute effort could
assume, but found it impossible to do so on the
body itself. I therefore had photographs taken
of a few people, chosen not from those whose
spines were very flexible, but from those whom
it was most convenient to photograph. One
of these persons, a woman aged thirty-two,
placed with the left shoulder against the wall,

---

* I have found that authors mention different parts
of the spine as enjoying most freedom of rotation, their
deductions being drawn from their ideas of the limit-
ing powers of the articulating processes. My belief,
founded on many observations on the living, is that
the freedom of movement is pretty evenly distributed.

was directed to bend the spine to the right as
much as she could without strain. On the
photograph of this position the transverse axis
of the pelvis was drawn, and a line at right
angles to it marks the straight position of the
spine: the curve from the top of the sacrum
to the vertebra prominens was then measured ;

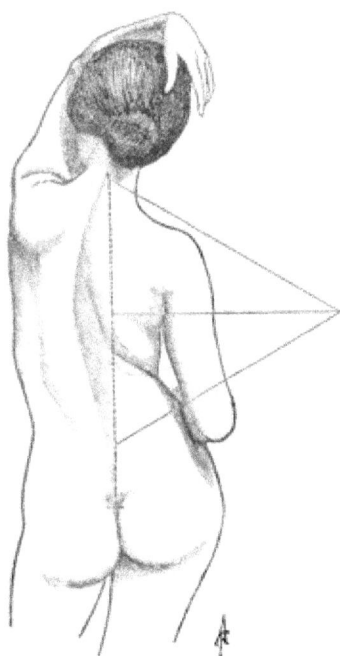

its length was 13·5 lines ; the radial distance
(we will suppose the curve circular) amounted
to twelve lines. On the body of the patient,

the length of the spine itself was eighteen
inches, therefore the radius of curve measured
sixteen inches. The dorsal and lumbar spine,
then, in ordinary individuals, and without
exertion, can bend laterally in a curve whose
radial distance is eight-ninths of its own
length. The curve, however, is not quite
circular; the greatest amount of bend takes
place between the seventh and tenth dorsal
vertebræ.

I also wished to study the conditions under
which the spine was placed in different actions
of the limbs and body. I therefore procured
a number of persons, chiefly artists' models, to
go through various movements with the back
naked. It does not seem advisable to tran-
scribe here my voluminous notes of these
experiments. Suffice it to say that in walking,
sitting down, and rising again, and lifting
even small weights, the spine bends from side
to side. As might be expected, motions of
the arms and shoulders influence chiefly the
upper part; movements of the lower limbs,
especially if the pelvis itself move, chiefly the
lower part, of the spine. The former move-

ments only affect the column when either
powerful or prolonged : for instance, a pound
weight may be held in the hand outstretched
without influencing the spine for a certain
time, but when fatigue commences the column
bends ; a greater weight will at the moment
of lifting cause bending of the column, produced in both instances by the spinal muscles
which lie at the opposite side to that which
carries the weight. Any movement which
shifts the weight of the body from one leg to
the other causes lateral flexion of the lumbar
and lower dorsal spine ; for instance, walking,
especially ascending a staircase, causes deviation to the right and left, in some persons as
high as the seventh dorsal, in others only to the
tenth dorsal vertebra. Whenever the weight
or movement be such as to cause more than
the slightest lateral bend, either in back or
loins, the other portion of the spine, loins,
or back, as the case may be, assumes a curve
in the contrary direction ; of this I shall have
to speak more fully in the sequel. With every
lateral movement a commensurate amount of
rotation is combined ; it does not appear

possible to bend the spine sideways without at the same time rotating the vertebræ to a certain extent.

The results of the above experiments show by mechanical measurement, that the spine is normally capable of a great amount of rotation, and of lateral flexion—a result which is in direct contradiction to the theory of a recent author, which, in order probably to justify the application of steel splints, would endeavour to prove the spine all but immobile. The writer in question says: "Horizontal rotation of the vertebræ exists only in the most limited degree, if, indeed, it can be said to exist at all, in the dorsal and lumbar regions" (Adams 'On Lateral Curvature,' p. 177). "The flexibility of the spine in a lateral direction is extremely limited" (p. 42). "The appearance of lateral flexibility is largely contributed to by the free ball-and-socket articulation of the hips and of the head" (p. 42). The author has thus come to the singular conclusion that the spine is all but a stiff column, from certain arguments about the direction and position of the articulating processes. The reasoning, however, is not very close; and we may be permitted to doubt its value when we encounter an explanatory diagram in which the axis of rotation is placed behind the tip of the spinous process, in which case rotation would indeed be limited. The axis of rotation between any two vertebræ is just behind the posterior edge of the bodies, *i.e.* in the spinal canal; and the spinal cord is placed close to that part of the vertebral bodies, *i. e.* in the axis of rotation, that pressure during such movement may be avoided.*

---

* I might in this place have omitted or modified the above references; but, since a short correspondence on this subject took place when these lectures appeared in the 'Lancet,' it seems to me more just to Mr. Adams to reproduce the matter exactly as it stood, and to annex the letters :—

" *To the Editor of* ' THE LANCET.'

"SIR,—I should be obliged by your permitting me to correct a misstatement of my views as to the flexibility of the spinal column in the dorsal and lumbar regions, made by Mr. Barwell, in the last number of 'The Lancet,' in a communication by him on Lateral Curvature of the Spine.

" After three fragmentary quotations, in the first of which an important part of the sentence is omitted without the usual sign (......) to indicate such omission, Mr. Barwell states that ' the author' (alluding to myself) ' has thus come to the singular conclusion that the spine is all but a stiff column.' Now, pro-

My measurements, however, may be taken
as indicating the normal movements of the

---

bably, very few of your readers would believe that I could hold
any such opinion; nor do I believe any one but Mr. Barwell
would accuse me of promulgating 'a theory which, in order probably to justify the application of steel splints, would endeavour
to prove the spine all but immovable.'

"Not content with a misstatement of my views, Mr. Barwell
thinks proper to add an unworthy motive for such views in
reference to the treatment adopted. I am at a loss to understand
Mr. Barwell's motives for making such an imputation in the
columns of 'The Lancet,' but will now ask any of your readers,
who may be sufficiently interested in the subject, to refer to my
recent work on 'Lateral and other Forms of Curvature of the
Spine,' from pp. 26 to 48, where they will find the subject of
horizontal rotation, and the flexibility of the spine in different
directions and in different regions, fully discussed, and the
observations of the highest recognised authorities referred to.

"As my object is simply to correct a misstatement, and not to
enter into any controversial discussion upon points in Mr. Barwell's communication, I beg to say that I shall not further reply
to any observations that may be made upon the subject.

" I am, Sir, yours, &c.,

" WILLIAM ADAMS.

" *Henrietta Street, Cavendish Square,*
        "OCT. 22nd, 1867."

" *To the Editor of* 'THE LANCET.'

"SIR,—While begging of you space for this short answer to
Mr. Adams' letter of last week, allow me, like him, to disclaim
any desire for controversy.

"I am very sorry that Mr. Wm. Adams should think he has
cause to complain that my quotations from his work on the
Spine are fragmentary, but fail to perceive how, in a short
paper, quotations from a large book can be otherwise. I have

spine. I desire to lay stress upon them because it will be found throughout the range

---

again carefully read the chapters from which the quotations were
taken, and, with the utmost liberality of interpretation, in the
new light which Mr. William Adams' letter provides, cannot
force upon the phrases any sense other than that which I have
already given them. Indeed, when a writer, describing 'horizontal rotation-movement of the spinal column,' says 'the extremely
limited extent of this movement' (p. 39); when he quotes and
agrees with another author who says that the 'oblique processes'
of the lumbar vertebræ 'prevent any twisting or spiral movement
whatever of the trunk upon the axis' (p. 40); and when,
throughout the chapter, the author constantly refers mobility to
the head, hips, and lumbo-sacral joints, rather than to the spine,—
I say, when an author writes thus, he must expect those of his
readers who understand the meaning of language to conclude
that he considers the spine very immobile. I do not at all understand how Mr. William Adams can imagine that I, in saying so,
have misinterpreted the meaning of the chapter to which he refers.

"Besides misrepresentation, Mr. Adams charges me with a
graver fault—namely, that I have accused him of 'unworthy
motives' in that he justifies his practice by his theory. Sir,
I believe that all practitioners prescribe medicines or appliances with reference to physiological or pathological doctrines
formed by themselves or taught in the schools. I hope we all
justify or endeavour to justify practice by theory. I may—
indeed I do—differ widely from the practice and theory of
Mr. Adams, and of the Orthopædic Hospital generally. Nevertheless, I have never written a single word reflecting on the
honour of its officers. It is not I, but Mr. Adams himself,
who suggests that 'unworthy motives' are required to justify
the application of steel supports to the vertebral column.

"I remain, Sir, your obedient servant,

"RICHARD BARWELL.

" *George Street, Hanover Square,*
"Nov. 12th, 1867."

Having

of pathology, that all deformities which progress slowly, and do not owe their origin to

---

Having done this justice to Mr. Adams, I must hold
the balance even for myself. The sentence which I
am accused of garbling, by omission of an important
part, occurs not in the chapter in which mobility or
rather immobility of the spine is discussed, but in
a much later section where, in controverting another
author, Mr. Adams sums up his ideas on the rotatory
power of the spine in one sentence thus :—" The direction and extent of the movements of the spine in the
different regions I have already fully discussed, and
satisfactorily shewn that horizontal rotation of the
bodies of the vertebræ—such as would be required to
give the spiral twist to the vertebral column—exists
only in the most limited degree, if indeed it can be said
to exist at all, in the dorsal and lumbar regions, where
lateral curvature commences, and in the latter is effectually prevented by the form and direction of the
oblique articulatory processes." My own feeling is
that no reader will imagine that the quotation in the
text alters the meaning of the sentence. I am the
more perplexed by Mr. Adams' letter, since the main
argument of his work appears to be that lateral flexibility and rotation of vertebræ are in health either
altogether absent or so insignificant that they can never
deviate into morbid postures or deformities, as witness :
—" Hence it is clear that when lateral curvature occurs in the lumbar region, which it does at least as
frequently as in the dorsal, it is not simply an exag-

destructive disease of bones and joints, consist at first only in the persistence of a posture which can naturally be assumed, it is in itself normal. After a time the position becomes exaggerated, *i. e.* it is in itself abnormal—such morbid posture may continue a certain time, according to the part affected, and age of the patient, without producing deformation of either bones or ligament, and until such alteration is produced the deformity is curable.

---

geration of a natural movement in this direction, as every anatomical provision is made to prevent lateral mobility " (p. 43).

CHAPTER II.

CAUSES OF DORSAL CURVATURE.

Each group of vertebræ—viz., cervical, dorsal and lumbar—may be affected by circumstances which produce in them a permanent curvature to one side. But when the first of these regions is the seat of such disturbance the malady is termed " wry neck," and, its production being peculiar, it is not included in the term of lateral curvature. The dorsal and the lumbar region only, consisting of seventeen vertebræ, are therefore to be included in the consideration of this malady. Let us commence with certain definitions and explanations, which will make our subsequent work easier.

A curvature is named right or left according as the convexity of the curve looks to the one or other side.

In every curvature the aberrant vertebræ twist, so that the anterior faces of their bodies look towards the convexity of the curve, the spinous processes to the concavity.

It very seldom happens that the spine assumes one simple lateral curve in the same direction from end to end.* On the contrary, there are at least two, in opposite directions; the upper one is called the dorsal curve, the lower, lumbar : dorso-lumbar would, however, be the more correct term, since it occupies the two or three lowest bones of the back, as well as those of the loins. Of these two curves, one is directly caused by some external circumstance, the other is only an indirect sequence, being produced by the necessity of restoring the balance disturbed by the curvature first set up. Hence the one is called primary, the other secondary or compensating.

The terms primary and secondary must be understood as referring only to the sequence

---

* Nearly all the examples I have seen of this condition were manifestly hysterical.

of causes; for, since the necessity of balance produces the secondary curve, it must arise simultaneously, or nearly simultaneously, with the primary one.

When more than two curves appear they are called multiple.

We will first consider curvature primarily dorsal as the more frequent and more important form; and in doing so must bear well in mind the three coincidences already specified, namely,—torsion of vertebræ, predominance of dorsal curvature to the right side, preference of the disease for the female sex. These peculiarities have not as yet been satisfactorily accounted for, and, since they are essential characteristics, I must beg the reader to dismiss as untenable any theory—my own among them—which does not fully explain their occurrence and their constancy.

The vertebræ and the ligaments of the spine are passive, and of themselves motionless objects. If any disease or alteration of shape caused them to deviate or to twist, such malady would after death be very apparent, and would long ere this have been distinctly

described in morbid anatomy ; but it would
be highly improbable, if not absolutely impossible, that the same side of the vertebræ, and
the same numerical vertebræ, should be so
constantly almost exclusively affected, that the
curve always influences the same bones. That
is to say, in a double curvature a straight line
from the last cervical vertebra to the middle
of the sacrum will cross the S shaped curve
once at the ninth dorsal vertebra, a few lines
below or above its spinous process, and this
whether the two curves be extreme or slight.
Therefore those who ascribe these curves to
a primary disease of bone or ligament are
bound to give some pathological history of
such malady, and to show cause why it
should affect not only particular bones, or
intermediate substances, but certain sides of
these particular parts, with such remarkable
constancy. We must then look outside the
spine for the causes of its curve, i. e., to the
forces which normally bend the spine in different directions, viz., to the muscles. The
muscular group classed together under the
name of erectores spinæ, being situated along

and parallel with the column, can have very little or no influence in rotating the dorsal portion of the spine.*

In the course of making the experiments detailed in the foregoing chapter, I was anxious to find what those forces might be which produce that normal rotation of the column whose amount I had so carefully measured. Somewhat unexpectedly, I found that rotation of the vertebræ in all the upper part of the column is effected by the serratus magnus, which when thin persons are under observation stands out during such action strongly and sharply. Let the reader consider the anatomical relations of this part. Two muscles (rhombodei major and minor) arising from the spine at the root of the neck and top of the back are inserted into the base of the scapula ; from this point the serratus spreads out fan-

* On the lumbar vertebræ, as we shall see in the sequel, their influence in this direction must be considerable ; if, however, dorsal curvature were attributable to this group, it is impossible to find any reason why it should so constantly affect one and the same side, and a group of vertebræ, nor why it should so predominate in one sex.

shaped, to be attached to the ribs from the
first to the ninth inclusive. For the particular

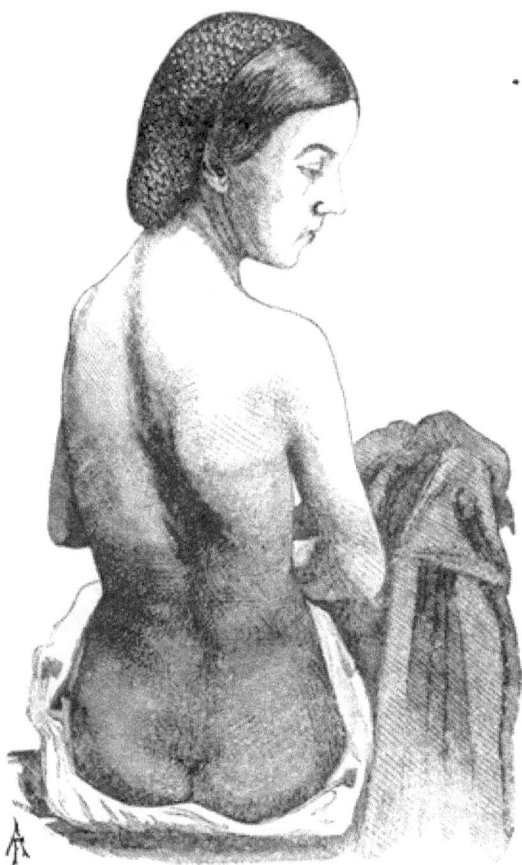

Rotating action of serratus.

action in question these muscles may be regarded as one broad fleshy layer, which,
arising from the upper part of the spine,

sweeps round and embraces the back and sides of the chest; and in this view the intervening base of the scapula is to be considered merely as an intersection, like the semilunar lines in the abdominal rectus. This muscular arrangement acts at great advantage in turning the upper part of the body on the pelvis; its base of attachment to the spine is small, its leverage short, that to the chest very large, and in contracting it draws the ribs of that side backward. Each rib, having attachment to the body, and also to the transverse process of vertebræ, becomes thus a lever of the second class, whose power arm is the length from the muscular attachment to its head, whose weight arm is the distance from head to tubercle; it is indeed a crow-bar very powerful to twist each vertebra on its own axis. This function of the rib is attested by the fact that when the serratus ceases to be inserted, the spinal attachment of the rib no longer affords a purchase for such action. In losing the double conjunction to body and transverse process, the lower ribs abrogate the arrangement of fulcrum and weight necessary to lever-like

action on the vertebræ, and at the same time
the serratus ceases to be attached to the ribs.

Now, let us consider the action of the serratus under another point of view. It has already been said, that only a very small portion
of the weight of the shoulder is supported
by the upper fibres of the trapezius, otherwise
its action on the head would have to be
counteracted by other muscles, which would
greatly interfere with the freedom and mobility
of the head and neck. Therefore the upper
angle of the scapula hangs to the spine by its
levator muscle ; but the outer angle, the
shoulder-joint and the arm, are supported by
the serratus, which, drawing the base and
lower angle of the shoulder outwards and forwards, keeps the outer angle (acromion and
shoulder) upwards and backwards. The
weight, therefore, of the shoulders, and of the
arms falls, through the medium of the serrati,
upon the ribs, and this weight tends to keep
them back—equally, of course, on both sides
of the chest if the arms be of equal weight.

The most important function, however, of
the serrati is respiratory ; they lift and draw

back the ribs on each side of the chest as far as the freedom at the joints permits, thus enlarging the cavity of the thorax. In forced inspiration this action is very marked; but man during quiet breathing hardly uses the muscle at all, his respiration being chiefly abdominal; woman's ordinary quiet breathing is, on the other hand, very much more pectoral, her chest and bosom rising constantly with each inspiration, even during sleep. In woman then, more than in man, the ribs are drawn backwards in inspiration—an action which would be equal on both sides of the chest if both lungs admitted the same quantity of air.

The hypothetical sentences at the end of the last two paragraphs are of importance. The arms are not of equal weight, nor are the lungs of the same size. A boy or youth, however, uses free exercise, swings his arms as he walks, and lolls and lounges about in all conceivable positions, thus giving variety to the manner in which the shoulders are supported; and, above all, he breathes chiefly by the diaphragm. The girl or young woman

takes less free exercise; in walking she lets
the arm hang almost motionless from the
shoulder, sits decorously upright, so that
the weight of the arms hangs all day long,
through the medium of the serratus magnus,
on the ribs; and, far more important, her
breathing is chiefly pectoral. Now let the
ribs be regarded, in the manner above described, as powerful levers, which, under the
sway of the serratus, can rotate the spine
should the one muscle act more powerfully
than its fellow; and consider the girl thus
circumstanced, with the right arm heavier
than the left, with the right lung more capa-
cious than the left, and it will be seen that
the serratus of the right side, being more
weighted and in stronger respiratory action
than its opponent, must of necessity rotate
the vertebræ to the left side. This explanation will at once account for the rotation of
vertebræ, and its prevalent direction. Moreover, a crucial proof, if I may use such a
term, is found in the fact that European
women, who by tight clothing round the
waist and abdomen increase their tendency to

pectoral respiration, are the frequent subjects
of lateral curvature; while among Hindoos,
Arabs, and others who use a loose form of
dress, such deformity is all but unknown.

Again, when part of one lung becomes, from
some local disease, unfit for its function, the
ribs covering that portion cease to move, and
are uninfluenced by those particular serrations
of the muscle. Therefore the corresponding
ribs of the sound side bulge backward, and
the cognate vertebræ become crooked. This
is not produced by contraction of the lung on
the diseased side (there is frequently rather
swelling than decrease in bulk), but from in-
action of the serratus over the affected spot;
the opposite parts of the muscle therefore
on the sound side must twist the vertebra,
since their action is unbalanced on the morbid
side of the chest. So accurate is this correspondence that we may fix upon the part of
lung most affected, by noting the ribs which
protrude on the sound side, and the locality of
the spinal deviation. In curvature from consumption, we find nearly always a high short
dorsal curve, as in a patient recently sent to

me by Dr. Cotton ; in pneumonia the curve is low and long, as I have had more than once occasion to remark in cases at the Charing-cross Hospital.*

It will, of course, be remarked that in this explanation I entirely change the sequence of causality. It is usually stated that the spine first curves laterally, then rotates, and in this latter movement, by dragging with it the ribs, deforms the chest. I affirm that the ribs are primarily drawn backwards, and, acting as levers, twist the vertebræ, which in consequence deviate from the right line—according to a simple mechanical law, and yielding to the new direction in which the erectors of the spine now act ; for in this rotated condition straightening the spine curves it naturally to the right, and in lateral curva-

---

* By no other method can we account for the fact that in pleurisy, when the size of the contents on one side of the chest is increased, and afterwards, when, the lung being bound down by adhesions, their size is diminished, we still have curvature in the same direction—i. e., from the diseased side ; the ribs on that side ceasing to move on respiration.

ture much of the sideways distortion is in
reality displaced extension.

In this etiology the different weight of the
two arms is not nearly of so much importance
as the peculiarities of the respiratory function ; yet even in the male subject the spine
is twisted slightly to the right so frequently
that such condition is by some regarded as
normal. A man, after the amputation of one
arm, acquires by the action of unequal weight
a certain amount of lateral twist, rarely sufficient to constitute a noticeable deformity.
When, however, a girl carries a weight constantly on one arm, its power in contorting
the spine becomes considerable, and we occasionally find nurse-girls become very crooked
from such cause. In these cases the lumbar
muscles on the other (the left) side of the
spine are found very much developed in consequence of increased action counterbalancing
the burden carried.* In such cases the compensatory lumbar curve is established simply

* This condition must be distinguished from mere
bulging of the parts through backward projection of
the transverse processes, as will be shortly explained.

for the sake of balance ; not so the secondary
curve in cases arising from respiratory causes.
The two forms are distinct, not only in causation but in form, and in the action of subtend-
ing muscles.

If the two causes (one-sided pectoral breathing and the influence of weight) be combined,
as is frequently the case, their distorting
power is very great; but the former is undoubtedly the more influential, and is continuous both night and day. European
women, as above stated, increase this peculiarity of thoracic breathing by wearing tight
petticoat-strings, corsets, and belts round the
waist ; also many plump girls, in desire to
restrain any unsightly, however blameless,
enlargement of the abdomen, frequently com-
press that part with belts or corsets, and thus,
by almost entirely checking the respiratory
movements of the abdomen, place themselves
in a position of dangerous facility for acquir-
ing dorsal curvature.

This leads me, even at the risk of future
repetition, to consider the grave cause of ob-
jection to the " spinal support" of orthopædy.

It is easily perceptible that there is great
difficulty, or rather impossibility, in fixing
around the pelvis a steel hoop so immovably
that a lever springing thereform can make
effective pressure on a protuberant portion
of the spine or ribs. In order, however, to
render the pelvic hoop of a spinal support
as little movable as possible, straps and bandages fastened upon the instrument encircle and
are tightly laced upon and around the abdomen. We have, however, just seen that excessively thoracic breathing of women (since
the right lung is larger than the left) is the
real and efficient cause of dorsal deformity.
Such exaggeration of woman's natural cha-
racter of respiration is produced chiefly or
entirely by tight swathing of the abdomen ;
for where this form of dress is not used, as
in hot climates, lateral curvature is a very
rare deformity. It is hardly necessary that
I should ask the reader to compare the cause
of lateral curvature with its prevalent treatment by an instrument which in every possible
way adds largely to the very root and origin
of the malady, by preventing abdominal move-

ment in breathing. Nor need attention be
called to the singular fact that tight rigid
stays have always, with justice, been regarded
as productive of lateral curvature; yet as
soon as a girl shows any inclination to that
deformity, she, under such treatment, is fixed
in stays, more tight, more heavy, and more
onerous than the most tyrannous devotee of
a barbarous fashion could invent. Yet we
must, in justice, state that in a certain small
number of cases these instruments have produced benefit—namely, in such as are caused,
not by the more usual respiratory conditions
above mentioned, but in that far smaller
number produced by distribution of weight
always to one side of the body. In such
cases the good is effected by the crutch-handle,
which relieves the serratus magnus of the
weight of the right shoulder. This may,
however, be effected, in the cases where it is
desirable, by means far simpler, and which
do not produce such restraint and so many
evils.

The production of the secondary curve
(lumbar) is somewhat different in each class

of case; for though, in either, two groups of muscles are called into play, viz., spinal and abdominal, yet the degree of their participation is not the same in both.

Let us first consider the formation of a lumbar curve consecutive to a weight-bearing dorsal curvature. A weight carried on the right arm alters in the figure the place of the centre of gravity; and in order to bring this within the points of support, the body is thrown over to the left side; the spine forms at first one simple curve to the right. This, as I have found by experiment on a number of individuals, is always the first new posture of the column, unless the weight be considerable in proportion to the person's strength. If the object be very heavy, or if the time for supporting it be prolonged, the spine, instead of bending thus simply, will form two curves; the upper one to the right will increase, and will be supplemented by another contrary curve in the loins.

Now, while the spine is straight as in infancy, the erectores spinæ muscles are placed at a mechanical disadvantage for

moving the bones in any direction, since a
cord running parallel to and in close contact
with a straight staff has less power in bending
that staff than if it ran in any other direction.
When, through the actions described in the
former chapter, the column assumes its antero-
posterior curves, the influence of the muscles
is improved, as far as backward and forward
movement is concerned; but still remain—
since the column in a lateral direction is
straight—in a disadvantageous posture for
producing sideways movement. But when
the spine, weighted as above described, has
become crooked (and this first step is chiefly
through the medium of abdominal muscles),
the erectores are in a better position for the
above action, and of course have most power
over those vertebræ which have chiefly deviated from the right line. We therefore
find, in all lateral curvatures of weight-bearing
origin, a line of strong muscular development
running from the back of the ilium to the
most aberrant vertebræ. This line is marked
in proportion to the weight carried and to the
rapidity with which the curve is formed. I

must, however, warn the unaccustomed observer against mistaking the projection formed
by prominent transverse processes in a rotated
lumbar spine for muscular enlargement.

The production of the compensating curve
in the much more frequent cases of respiratory
origin is very different. In normal breathing
inspiration is produced by descent of the diaphragm, together with relaxation of the abdominal muscles and protrusion of the belly.
When such movement is restrained by any
pressure over the abdomen, this relaxation is
prevented, but the same cause does not prevent—indeed it rather abets—constant contraction of the abdominal muscles. The spine,
however, twisting to the right, relieves the
tension of the left side, while that on the right
is increased, not merely by this twist, but by the
respiratory elevation of the ribs. Thus upon
these right ribs two forces act at an angle to
one another: one from the pelvis drawing
them down, the other from the spine drawing
them upwards and backwards. These forces
balance each other, since during life there is
no alteration of the costo-spinal angle; but

the pelvis, in its relationship to the trunk, is a
fixed point, the spine a movable one.   Hence,
although the former force does not change the
posture of the ribs on the spine, it draws ribs
and spine *en masse, i. e.* the whole trunk down
to the right hip-bone, causing the loins to
bend chiefly at or near the second lumbar
vertebra : such, at least, is the point at which
in practice we find the greatest aberration.
If we consider this subject in a more mechanical point of view, the problem may be placed
thus:— Upon each rib two forces act, at an
angle to each other, and the resultant movement must be in a line within the angle. Since
the rib itself does not move on the spine, the
forces are even, therefore this line of motion
must bisect the angle ; and, of course, the point
of movement must be where that line inter-
sects the next jointed part of the body.   The
annexed rough diagram represents, on the
right side, the lines of force of the serrati and
external oblique with the bisecting lines of
movement.   Now, if these measurements be
made on the subject, and the lines carefully
drawn, it will be found that they all converge

to a space between the first and third lumbar
vertebræ. Hence, in cases of respiratory
origin, unless far advanced, we find on the

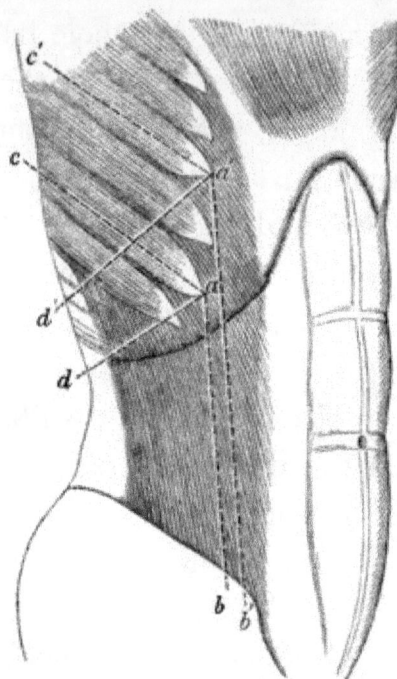

a b, and c' a b', the angle of serratus and lateral oblique at seventh and
ninth ribs; a d, and a d', the bisecting line.

left loin no line of strong muscular development present in the weight-bearing curve;
but on the right side we find exaggerated
muscular marking about the side and flank,

with—what will most strike the unaccustomed observer—a twisting of the umbilicus. These diagnostic signs will require especial consideration in the sequel.

CHAPTER III.

CAUSES OF LUMBAR CURVATURE.

IN order to trace the simpler etiology of
lumbar curves, I would remind the reader
of those parts in the first chapter, which refer
to the normal movements of the spine in different actions of the body. The erect human
figure has but two points of support, and in loco-
motion the weight is thrown alternately from
one to the other : thus a certain shifting of the
centre of gravity takes place, so as to bring it
over the right and left foot by turns. Such
movement occurs even in walking along level
ground ; and, besides this, the pelvis twists a
little with every step, so that first one side and
then the other is advanced, and the side projected forward is at the same time lifted.
These conditions necessitate certain movements of the spine, which may be felt, as

before stated, in some as high as the seventh dorsal, in others only to the tenth or eleventh dorsal. The highest movements of the column are, *cæteris paribus*, to be found in women, a fact which is, I believe, attributable to their greater breadth of pelvis.

Since the actions of limbs and pelvis alternate, so must the spine move from side to side, producing those exquisite curves of graceful action which the Greeks so wonderfully understood. These, I say, take place even in walking over a level space; they are, of course, increased in such actions as ascending a staircase, or more unevenly, but to a larger extent, in passing over broken ground. Such curves (without, however, the pelvic twist) can be well observed in the back of one sitting on a prancing horse or sailing over a chopping sea; but it is most thoroughly to be observed by seating an individual, sideways and barebacked, on a plank contrived to rock on a fitting support placed under the centre of gravity. An observer standing behind the subject of experiment will see alternating undulations of the spine, as depicted in the

E

accompanying diagram. If the whole spine
remained at right angles to the pelvis when

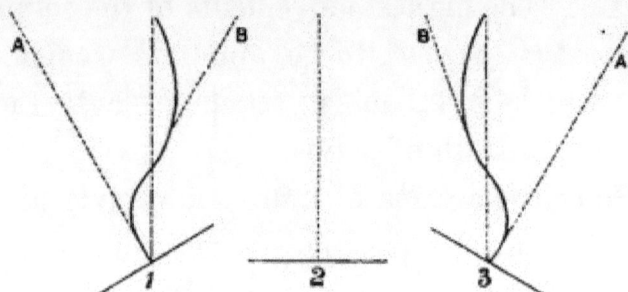

2, The horizontal position. 1 and 3, Rocking to right and left. The dotted
lines, A A, the direction of lower lumbar vertebræ. B B, The direction of
dorso-lumbar spine. The central dotted line, a perpendicular. The dark
lines, curves of spine.

its transverse axis became oblique (1 and 3,
A A), the line of gravity would fall outside
the support; therefore the spine bends to the
right. Moreover, since the centre of gravity
lies so low in the body, this bend must be
sharp. If the upper part of the trunk followed the direction of the loins (1 and 3, B B),
the balance would be over-corrected; hence
the dorsal portion must assume a contrary
curve. These movements, though owing to
the necessities of balance, are of course produced entirely by muscular action.

All observant people are aware that they
very seldom see an individual standing with

the weight equally distributed between the
two feet—*i. e.*, with a perpendicular spine
erect upon a horizontal pelvis. On the contrary, the ordinary standing position is a little
crooked, the weight is thrown more on one
leg than on the other, the pelvis is more or
less oblique, and there is a commensurate bend
therefore in the lumbar spine, to which the
second and third vertebræ chiefly contribute,
while a long consecutive curve is formed in
the dorsal region. Now it is evident that if
any peculiarity cause this pelvic obliquity,
with its chain of consequences, to occur
always on the same side, the position will by
degrees become more marked, and ultimately
permanent. This influence is, of course, most
potent in cases, where some malady of the
lower limbs produces a continual inclination of
the pelvis. Thus an individual with a varous
foot, an anchylosed knee, or contracted hip,
being forced to curve the back in a manner
compensating the pelvic obliquity, will, after
a time, most certainly acquire a morbid bend
of the spine towards the lower side of the
pelvis; and although, in the early part of

the case, such curve is annulled when the
pelvic obliquity is for the moment artificially
corrected, or when the patient lies down, yet
it will after a time become permanent, and
does not thus disappear.

From this statement it becomes evident that
bad habits of walking or position, which render the pelvis oblique, will also produce
lumbar curvature with a rapidity propor-
tionate to the inveteracy of the habit. The
potency of a cause which at first glance
would appear so slight will be more readily
appreciated if the attachment of muscles supporting the spine on the pelvis be considered.
These are, besides the abdominal muscles—
whose power has already been mentioned,—
the *erectores spinæ*, the quadratus lumborum
and the psoas : the mere supporting action of
the two first is evident ; it will be necessary to
refer to them again, but just now I desire
to call attention to the last. The psoas has,
as we have seen, very considerable influence
in producing the anterior curve of the lumbar
spine, through the tension exerted on them by
the erect posture of the thighs ; the muscle

runs from these vertebræ to the back part of
the inner side of the femur, in such wise that
all movements of the limb, except, possibly,
ab- and adduction—that is to say, extension,
flexion, inward and outward rotation — all
either extend or relax this muscle. A tempo-
rary movement of this sort, a position assumed
casually and for a time, will not affect a spine,
supported as it is by other muscles; but a constant and overweening posture is less guarded
against, and the parts gradually yield. It is
not at the moment of active force that malposture is produced, but during the relaxation of
an ill-regulated repose. Thus other postures,
besides those causing obliquity in the transverse
direction of the pelvis, as sitting cross-legged,
have their effect in producing a lumbar curve;
indeed all positions which twist the pelvis and
cause unequal tension of the thighs are especially prone to produce this condition.*

---

* Three cases have come under my notice, in which
I could distinctly trace the origin of lumbar curve to
this position. Its powerful effect has three causes :—
One, that the thigh crossed (say the left) is placed
higher than the other, and rotated outwards (relaxing

All such tricks in young growing people
should be checked, but more especially in
girls, who, leading generally a less active life,
are more exposed to the influence of such
habits, and whose greater width of pelvis
adds to the danger. The deformity comes on
so very slowly, as rarely to be detected by
daily companions, but is generally first observed by a dress-maker or dancing-master,
who points out that one or the other hip
protrudes; for while in dorsal curves prominence of a shoulder first attracts attention, the
prominent hip is the first observed defect in
those affected with lumbar curve.

In the above description all reference to
rotation of vertebræ has been omitted, that
the succession of events might with greater
ease be followed: nevertheless rotation is part
and parcel of this malady—one of the neces-

---

the left psoas); another, that the knee is advanced in
front of the right one—*i. e.*, the pelvis is twisted; a
third, the weight is thrown chiefly on the right haunch.
All these aid in producing curvature to the right,
leaving the weight of the body constantly more on
one leg than on the other.

sary conditions of the muscular action which induces
the curve.

The adjoining diagram
shows the spine, with its normal antero-posterior curves
very carefully reduced to
scale. The erectores spinæ
is not to my mind well described in English anatomical
works, they do not define
the differences in mass of
various parts of this muscle
as they really exist. The incurvation of the loins, from
close to the skin to the lumbar
transverse process, is filled up
by a muscular mass, which
in a grown man is about
two inches thick. Most of
the fibres run forwards, and
more or less upwards, and
gain insertion in the transverse processes; others, the
more superficial ones, pass

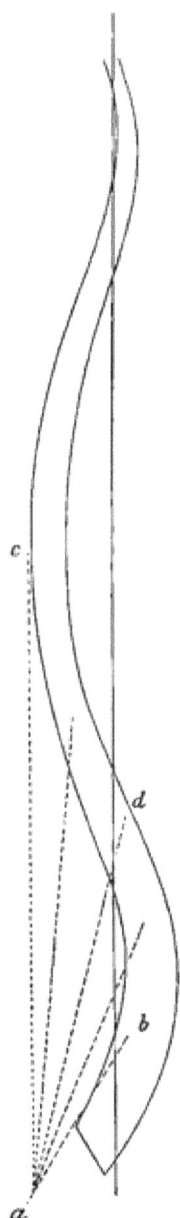

A view of the normal curves of the spine seen from the right side, and showing the attachments of lumbar muscles in section. Angle *b*, *a*, *d*, the lumbar. Angle *c*, *a*, *d*, the dorsal part of the muscle.

directly upwards, and, dividing into two portions, are fixed, the outer part, to the ribs, the
inner to the dorsal transverse processes. Thus
a longitudinal section through the body on the
plane of the tips of the transverse process
would discover the muscle as a fan-shaped
mass; it will readily be seen, from the above
diagram, that the lower or lumbar portion
must act as a rotator, the upper simply as an
extensor.

It cannot be too strongly impressed upon
the minds of those unaccustomed to examine
these cases, that the rotation always takes
place so that the fronts of the vertebræ face
towards the convexity of the curve : in consequence of this the transverse processes on
that convexity may be felt with more or less
distinctness according to the amount of bend ;
and, in thus rising from the depths to the
surface of the loins, they lift with them
the muscles and other soft parts, while on the
other side the transverse processes sink deeply
towards the abdomen ; and the lumbar muscles
sink with them, so that losing their hard support, they become soft and doughy. This con-

dition on the convex side has been mistaken
for violent or spastic contraction of muscle; and
the view has led to sundry infelicitous errors
in theory and practice. For instance, these
muscles have been cut, and, singular to relate,
M. Guerin, who originated this operation, has
cut muscles sometimes on the convex, sometimes on the concave side of the spine with,
according to his published writings, equally
brilliant results : indeed, this operation has
been revived at one of the many special
Hospitals. It is a pity that the strong con-
demnation passed upon it by a commission
of the most celebrated Parisian surgeons has
not deterred orthopædists from this justly
condemned procedure. Its future fate can
be foreseen with only too great facility, it is
written in the pages of the past. While
subcutaneous myotomy and tenotomy were
still new, its employment was in Paris transferred from the limbs to the trunk, and a certain number of cases suffered under the knife;
while the debility thus induced permitted the
scaffoldings to work with greater ease, the
operator, and perhaps his patients, buoyed

themselves with hopes that a cure was hatch-
ing—the cases were published with considerable parade and flourish, and a few more
induced to undergo myotomy. Then came a
time when some ventured to express distrust
of these results. That feeling gradually
gained ground, and after a time it was found
that at a period when, if a cure had been
effected, the patient might have dispensed
with mechanism, a stronger support instead
of a slighter one was needed: the back
became weaker, and collapsed when the irons
were removed, at last was scarcely able, even
with strong instruments, to uphold the trunk
at all. Then these cases were not so much
paraded; the Academy pronounced a con-
demnation of the procedure; and the whole
thing has been quietly interred, until in these
latter days, when its ineffectual ghost haunts
us once again.

CHAPTER IV.

DIAGNOSIS OF DIFFERENT CURVES.

WE have seen that a broad and marked distinction between a curve primarily lumbar, and one primarily dorsal, lies in the fact that in the former a prominent hip, in the latter a prominent shoulder, is first observed ; that is, such changes give rise to the most marked symptom of each malady. Thus, though a dorsal curve very rapidly, perhaps instantaneously, calls forth a lumbar, and the primarily lumbar is closely followed by a secondary dorsal, yet the peculiar first alteration remains characteristic till, at all events, a late period, and not unfrequently throughout the case ; and this peculiarity is not the lateral sinuosity of the column, but the twist backwards of parts on the convex side of the spine, or, if it be very early in the case, on the side which will become convex.

Thus, if the surgeon be about to examine a patient with the desire of finding out whether or no the spine be crooked, he will be judicious in directing attention rather to the parts above named than to the line of the spinous processes, for the following reasons :—When, in the commencement of the malady, the vertebræ begin to deviate, they do so in two manners—rotation and lateral movement. Now, the tip of the spinous process—which, until there is considerable displacement, is the only bit of the bone we can feel—is that very part which in rotating moves most away from the side to which lateral displacement tends : therefore there is a stage in the condition, when the tips of these processes will lie in a straight continuous line, and yet the vertebræ will have been considerably displaced. But, if we direct our research to the parts at the side of the spine, we find that these, be they ribs or lumbar and pelvic bones, have been so displaced that, under good auspices of lighting, the eye will detect the want of symmetry, or a practised hand will distinguish the variation of level. Some stress is laid upon the mode of lighting,

because in an ordinary window light any
horizontal gradual protuberance or undula-
tion can hardly be detected; but, with a perpendicular light, the shoulder in the one class,
the hip, or rather haunch, in the other class
of curve, receives on its prominence a strong
ray, and throws a long shadow under its
elevation. I have the advantage of possessing
two consulting-rooms, and have found that an
amount of torsion so slight as to be not at all
or doubtfully perceptible in the one light was
unmistakably evident in the other. The fact
of unsymmetrical shading of the torso must
provisionally be considered as sufficiently indicative of a spinal curve. We shall speak
of more conclusive symptoms in the sequel.
Instances of this condition will be found in
the annexed engraving for the one form, and
in the cut at p. 68 for the other.

After having decided on the existence of
a spinal curve, the next points for examination are these :—firstly, is it primarily dorsal
or primarily lumbar? and, if the former, to
which class of dorsal curves does the distortion belong? The former question must be

answered by observation concerning relative
protuberance of the hip or of the posterior
pectoral walls. I will describe the differential
diagnosis as shortly as possible, since the
peculiarities of each case must be again discussed in their special description. The mere
projection of the scapula is comparatively a
late symptom in dorsal curve : previous to
its appearance a certain bulging beneath and
outside the angle of the blade-bone becomes
evident. In lumbar curve, again, the lateral
projection of the hip—that which alters the
mere outline of the figure—is later than a
posterior projection of the innominate bone,
marked by protuberance backward of the
parts lying just outside the sacro-ilac joint;
while the figure above this, though it may
not have altered to the view, will be found
by touch harder on one side of the spine than
on the other—a difference resulting from the
unsymmetrical positions of the transverse processes, not from muscular transformations.
Diagnosis in all disease is simple enough, if
strongly marked types of malady be assumed;
the skill of an observer is shown in his power

of distinguishing in early stages where the typical conditions, though present, are still only in part developed. Now, in all cases of dorsal curve, the mere lateral undulations of the bones of the spine will not afford any ground for diagnosis; but the variations in collateral parts give ample means for distinguishing the forms, under such conditions as I have named. In the very earliest stages, the costal prominence backward of a dorsal curve is unaccompanied by any pelvic change—nor in an equally early stage of lumbar curve, is the backward gluteal projection combined with any pectoral alteration; but these, with certain others hereafter described, will indicate the presence of a lateral curve before the line of the spinous processes has deviated to any appreciable extent. In later stages a curve primarily dorsal will be accompanied by lateral prominence of the other hip, but never by the peculiar backward prominence above described.

The diagnosis between lumbar and dorsal curvature being now formed, it will be desirable to point out the peculiarities of each; and first of the dorsal curve.

The backward projection of the scapula is, I have said, a rather late symptom, and it will be well to explain its occurrence. The first motive of a dorsal curve is, as has been shown, over-action in one serratus,—*e.g.*, the right, which draws back, and a little upwards, the ribs; it follows that inequality in the walls of the chest will be an early sign. Moreover, since a slight twist in such short and such well-covered bones as the vertebræ can hardly be detected, but becomes very evident in such long levers as the ribs, it follows that, although from their anatomical connections both parts must rotate at the same time, yet the ribs by their length will act as indices, and enable us at once to detect an amount of rotation not evidenced by the shorter bones. In their backward progress the ribs begin to press upon the soft parts which separate them from the scapula, and these all yield, to a certain extent, before the pressure becomes sufficient to raise the bone itself: thus in the earlier stages the scapula may still be in

normal position. Be it also remembered that
the shoulder is very movable, and it frequently
happens that in making examination of a
young woman we shall find, in spite of all
possible care to keep the arms in position and
the back upright, that sometimes one, sometimes the other bladebone will project more
than its fellow, on account of some irregular
action of muscles induced by the exposure to
the air of parts usually covered, a sense of
shyness, or impress of the surgeon's finger.
Such impress is necessary : for, while examination by the eye is highly essential,
we must also use touch ; feeling not only for
the projection of the ribs of transverse processes on the right side, and their depression
on the left, but also for the line of the spinous
processes. It will hardly be necessary, in this
advanced stage of our investigations, to repeat
that the axis of rotation lies just at the
posterior margin of the vertebral bodies, and
that the tips of the spinous processes being
twisted to the left may still be in a straight
line, although the spine itself will have deviated considerably ; but it will be well to

F

point out a peculiarity which, as far as I
know, has not been noticed. There is in the
skin of the back a mesial line, or broad raphé,
very plainly marked by absence of hair-follicles
and gland-ducts, and by the opposed direction
of those structures on each side. This line,
while the back is straight, lies over the spinous
projections; but when these latter deviate
they glide beneath the skin, and may wander
considerably from the mesial line without
drawing the raphé with them. Therefore it
is not sufficient to examine by sight alone, for
the superficial marking will be sure to mislead
the eye as to the position of deeper parts. If
the case be advanced beyond the very earliest
stage, the surgeon will be able to feel the tips
of the spinous processes on one side (under the
circumstances postulated on the right side) of
this line, and about an inch further the transverse processes begin—as the curve advances—
to be perceptible, or, at the least, there will be
the hardness produced by their retrogression
towards the surface.

Although it is desirable to avoid examining
the front of the figure as much as possible,

yet it is well to know the changes which take place. These are very early, and, since they depend upon torsion to the right side, are very simple. In normal conditions, a straight line—a piece of cord, for instance—laid upon the middle of the first sternal bone, and passed between the thighs, should bisect the breast-bone, the xiphoid cartilage, and the umbilicus, running over a well-defined abdominal raphé. In lateral curvature, a line similarly placed on the upper piece of the sternum, and held in the same way, no longer coincides with these mesial parts of the body; but the breast-bone slants away from it to the right, the xiphoid cartilage and the umbilicus lie altogether to its right. The part most deviated is the tip of the ensiform cartilage : thus the cord forms the base of an obtuse triangle, the sides which subtend the blunt angle being formed by the mesial line of the sternum above, and by the linea alba of the abdomen below. Coincident with this deviation are certain changes in the apparent size of the left and right chest : we have seen that the right ribs are drawn back, and the vertebræ, by their rota-

F 2

tion, throw the left ribs forward ; thus, viewed from the front, the chest presents an appearance just the contrary to its aspect from

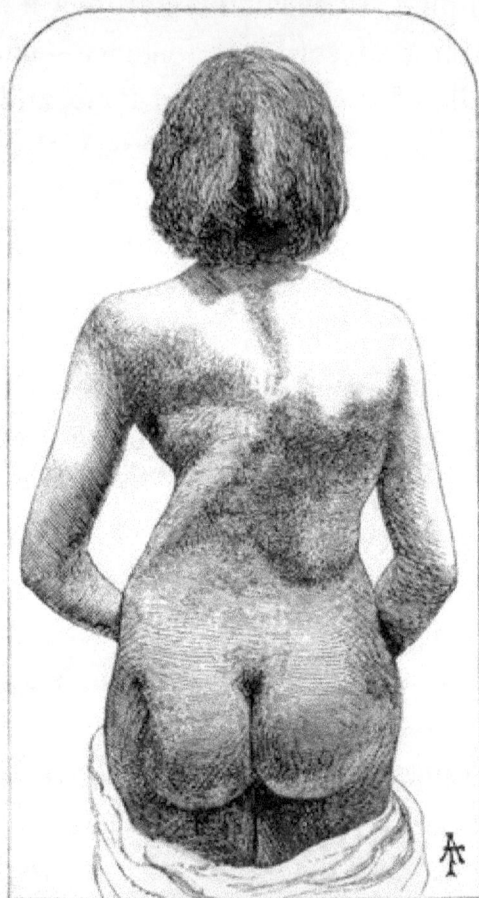

The patient had a far advanced respiratory curvature; for which she had worn instruments of considerable weight for some years. Note the absence of any projection of lumbar muscles on the left side; the line of light running from the ilium is simply the edge of the body and of the hollow from sinking forward of the ribs; it springs from the ilium far outside the erector spinæ.

behind, viz.—the right side appears small and shrunken, the left prominent and on a plane further forward than its fellow.

A great aid to diagnosis, or rather, let me say, a reliable means of confirming or negativing conclusions drawn from subtle changes of form, is to be found in the rotation measurer, which I have already described. After having studied the results of experiments with this instrument on the healthy subject, I expected, when first applying it to patients, to find that rotation to the side towards which the spine curves (let us suppose the right) would be greater than in the opposite direction. I soon found, however, that this notion was directly contrary to the truth : rotation to the right side is decreased ; while to the left that power is relatively, I believe often absolutely, increased. The reason of this is not far to seek : it lies in the facts that the bones have already performed a certain part of their possible rotatory journey to the right, and the chief muscle for this action (serratus magnus) has, in a measure, done its work. Torsion to the left, on the other hand, replaces the bones and ligaments, and the muscle itself is not merely in a state of quiet, but is in such a position as renders the range of its action larger than usual. Accordingly, in all cases of lateral curvature, the index of my instrument indicates to right and left a difference in degrees, whose number corresponds with the extent of the curvature. A small margin of difference often, indeed generally, occurs in perfectly straight spines; but this surplusage is nearly always to the right, and does not exceed five degrees; such difference, especially in that direction, may be discarded.*

Since, then, the rotation measurer marks a greater or less amount of difference as the case is more or less severe, the instrument becomes of great value as an index of success in treatment; since if the patient be improving the discordance diminishes, and in-

---

* We must here except the cases in which the ordinary orthopædic supports have been worn. Spines subjected to that treatment are usually stiff, and the muscles much wasted, so that they rotate but very little and unevenly; therefore no information can be gained from their action.

creases if she be getting worse. Thus I shall in the sequel mark the progress of certain related cases by a diary of rotation, to show the precision of its indications.

When the mere existence of a dorsal curvature has been detected, we must then, in order to apply treatment aright, distinguish the class of curve to which the case belongs, and must primarily divide these distortions into two sets—the curve from respiratory causes, and the curve of weight-bearing origin.

In the *Weight-bearing* class of cases I have observed but one sort—it is that which has been already in part described. The curve occupies the upper three-fourths of the dorsal region, and the return for the compensatory curve commences with the lower fourth. A straight line—a silken thread, for instance—stretched between the last cervical vertebra and the middle of the sacrum crosses the double curve *once* at the ninth dorsal vertebra. The most aberrant bones are the fifth dorsal to one side, the second lumbar to the other.*

---

* These numbers may not be absolutely rigid. but are remarkably uniform.

A well-marked rounded eminence of muscular contraction runs upward from the back part of the ilium to the most aberrant vertebra. Most of these curves are to the right; but as *all* respiratory curves, lung-disease being absent, are to the right (save in the very exceptional instances of visceral transposition), a curve primarily dorsal to the left, if the breathing apparatus be sound, and if the heart beat on the left side of the chest, may be certainly set down as weight-bearing. There is to be traced in almost all of these cases some history of hard work, generally at an early age, as constantly carrying an infant or other weight, &c. By far the larger proportion of this sort of curve belongs, therefore, to the working class. They are less frequent, and for that and other reasons less important, than the respiratory curves. They are also more easily cured if the individuals can so far alter their habits as to relieve the overworked muscles. This concession is, however, in that class of persons with difficulty obtained.

Of the *Respiratory Curves* there are two sorts: the one arising from external causes,

restraint of abdominal breathing, and even
certain bad habits; the other originating in
some malady of the lung and appendices.
This latter class of cases is not only very
interesting, but of great moment, and it will
be well to draw attention strongly to certain
important features, especially on that view of
the lung malady on which, as a surgeon, I am
authorised to speak—viz., of the form, state,
and position of curves which should lead us to
anticipate internal disease.

This class of curve is then always (save in
the extremely rare cases of transposed viscera)
to the right; it occupies, like that from weight-
bearing, the upper three-fourths of the dorsal
spine, and the point of greatest aberration
falls on the same vertebræ. It is barely possible to distinguish between the two classes by
the mere form of the curve alone; yet, since
differences exist in its aspects, and as certain
extraneous characteristics are obvious, the distinction can always be made. The upper limb
of the curve is more marked, the lower less so,
and both are less straight—that is to say, suppose the fifth dorsal vertebra at a given dis-

tance of lateral deviation in the weight-bearing
curves, the lines of spinous processes running
upward and downward from this vertebra are
almost straight, so that it seems to be in an
angle; in the respiratory form the curve,
though equal in amount, is more evenly distributed over the nine upper dorsal bones.
There is no line of strong muscular development running up from the back of the ilium;
the secondary curve is, in proportion, less
severe.

Curves of internal origin assume a variety
of shapes, from the gradual long curve occupying all, or nearly all, of the dorsal region, to
the well-marked short and sudden aberration
of two or three vertebræ occurring anywhere
between the first and the tenth. These latter,
particularly if they be high, are generally
connected with tubercle of the lung. Pneumonia induces, as a rule, the low long curve
which, even when the functions of the lung
have been restored, continues for a long time,
perhaps permanently, after the attack has
passed off. Pleurisy produces several forms of
curve, but chiefly a high curve, longer and less

sharp than the consumptive curvature. In
my second paper I hinted at the etiology of
these deformations ; they do not arise from
contraction on the diseased side, but from the
fact that when any portion of the lung becomes
unfit to perform its office, or when disease
renders such performance painful, the rib or
ribs, over that part of the organ cease to move,
while those on the other side continue, under
the sway of the serratus, to act unopposed
upon the vertebræ, and twist them round. If
we consider the great power of the ribs as
levers, the length of their power-arm, the
shortness of their weight-arm, we shall com-
prehend the sensitiveness of the spine to their
action.

In the course of these papers a cause which
is often given for lateral curve has been omitted—viz., " *position* ;" and this has been done
because *position* of the spine itself—*i. e.*, different habits of sitting or lying—does not often
in my experience produce this deformity. Position of pelvis and thighs is, as we have seen,
the efficient cause of curvatures primarily
lumbar ; position of the ribs of those primarily

dorsal. The shoulder and arm are, as a rule, in such varied movement that curvature very rarely depends on their posture; nevertheless, I shall immediately give a striking example to the contrary.

In considering the causes of these changes in form of dorsal curve, we must dismiss from our minds all inconclusive and unsatisfactory theories concerning its origin in spastic con-traction of muscles—in paralysis of respiratory function, in softening or inflammation of bones, intervertebral substance, &c., and ac-cept entirely the simple, and, as it appears to me, adequate doctrine taught in these chapters—that in the sequence of causes for dorsal curvature torsion precedes lateral devia-tion—that none of the spinal muscles proper are capable of producing such rotation; but that the lever-like arrangement of the ribs, enabling the serrati to turn the trunk in either direction, gives to those muscles, when uni-laterally and unduly exerted, the power of inflicting on the vertebræ a permanent twist, which of necessity is followed by lateral devia-tion. Perhaps, however, some of my readers,

unaccustomed to watch the power of muscles
in producing deformity, will scarcely estimate
the extreme sensitiveness of the spine to the
exaggerated action of one serratus. Let the
following case illustrate this point :—

Mr. ———, aged nineteen, came to me on the 9th of
February, 1867, with a far advanced dorsal curve to
the right. He was by no means weakly, but on the
other hand muscular, being used to strong exercise,
more especially with the dumb-bells. Rotation was
very marked, the ribs and the lower angle of the
scapula projecting very much backward : but there was
something very peculiar in the distortion ; it bore,
markedly, all the characteristics of a weight-bearing
curve, with the exception of its most prominent feature
—the strong development of the left sacro-lumbalis
and longissimus dorsi. It is true that he confessed to
using the dumb-bells rather more with the right than
with the left hand ; but in all my previous cases I had
always found such or similar work produce with the
curve the muscular elevation so often mentioned. The
condition was, to my mind, so anomalous that I re-
examined all my minute records, my photographs, and
my theory of lateral curvature. On his second visit I
observed this peculiarity of attitude : he always stood
with the right hand placed far back on the hip or on
the loins, and threw his elbow as far back as possible.
I kept him with me as long a time as I could spare,
and standing as much as possible. He maintained constantly this attitude ; and, on questioning him, I found

it was habitual. Thus, then, was my difficulty not
only solved, but a singular proof added to my observations. This position, by throwing back the base of
the scapula, caused the serratus to drag upon the ribs,
and not only the absence of an extra burden, but the
fact of his supporting the weight of the trunk on the
right hand, precluded the extra development of the left
erectores spinæ.

A few less well-marked dorsal curves, produced by position, doubtless occur — such
postures, for instance, as sempstresses, book-
stitchers, &c., assume, cause occasionally long
and slight dorsal deviations; but the generality
of curvatures owing their origin to posture are
undoubtedly lumbar.

Although the differential diagnosis between
lumbar and dorsal curvature has been shortly
and succinctly given, it will be desirable to
recur to certain of the signs of lumbar curvature, and to enforce the distinction with
greater minuteness. As the primarily dorsal
curve commences above, in posterior pro-
cession of the ribs, so the primary lumbar
curve begins in a similar displacement of
other parts, viz., of certain portions of the
pelvis. Let us, *exempli gratiâ*, assume that

the curvature under examination be lumbar to the right—that is to say, such a curve is about to appear; but, long previously to any absolute change in the spinal bones, we observe an alteration in neighbouring parts, revealed, as already stated, under a perpendicular light. In all these cases it is of the utmost importance to obtain the earliest reliable diagnostic sign of the morbid condition, and I would strongly impress upon my readers that the mere lateral protrusion of the hip, whereby the deformity is first recognised by parents, dressmakers, or other unskilled observers, is in reality a late symptom. A peculiar backward projection of the pelvis, *i. e.*, of the haunch, or, to be more precise, of the parts just outside the sacro-iliac joint, on the side towards which the spine is about to, or has become convex, is the earliest symptom.

This change, though more marked in some cases than in others, is, in my experience, always present in a curve primarily lumbar: it may be detected long before lateral projection supervenes, while lateral deviation of the spine can hardly, or not at all, be recognised.

A woodcut will be found at p. 119, which, chiefly intended to show a form of bandage, has been carefully drawn in well chosen light and shade, and therefore gives with considerable accuracy this diagnostic projection. It is not, however, to be supposed that this one symptom is to be accepted as the integral diagnosis, although it is in the earliest stage all that is perceptible to the eye; if, however, we examine by touch the parts just above the pelvis, and contiguous to the spinous processes, we find that on one side—that of the protuberant pelvis—the parts will be harder, more resilient than the other; a little later, the transverse processes will be felt on deep pressure, and, as they become more perceptible, the line of the spine gradually yields and curves towards the indurated side.

CHAPTER V

SIGNS OF CURABILITY.

BEFORE passing on to consider what sort of treatment will best befit the conditions whose origin has been in the foregoing chapters explained, it will be well to examine what circumstances would in any given case lead us to view it as curable or the reverse. To gain a clear insight into these peculiarities the reader must dismiss from his mind all those inconclusive theories which have been already shortly examined. It has been shown (p. 4) that the origin of lateral curvature cannot possibly be in diseases of vertebral bodies, nor of intervertebral substances, neither in weakness, nor in spastic contraction of spinal muscles; since, under such circumstances, we should find preference of this malady neither for one side nor for one sex. Nevertheless an

G

advocate for cutting the spinal muscles has recently insisted on this theory, because he has found in certain autopsies the *erectores spinæ* of one side degenerated. He appears to forget or ignore that all muscles, partly or entirely thrown out of gear, and out of use, are by the imposed restraint subject to fatty or to fibrous degeneration, according as the abnormal position produces tightness or looseness of their fibres. It is not enough, when conducting an autopsy, to observe a change; it is also necessary to distinguish between primary and secondary metamorphoses, and to know the difference between cause and effect.

A muscle, in strong and active, even exaggerated use, like the arm of a blacksmith, does not degenerate, but grows. Therefore the overworked serratus of one side, would (if we could make such an experiment) weigh more than the other. By this overaction the spine is twisted, the spinal muscles are thereby so placed that they in great measure, and after a time almost entirely, lose their normal action—they degenerate, therefore; those on the convex side become fibrous, those on the concave fatty.

The preponderance of muscular action on one side of the body, which produces lateral curvature, is not an action morbid in itself, like a spastic or convulsive contraction (supposing that such action can exist in a chronic state at all), it is simply an overaction imposed upon the muscles by extrinsic conditions already discussed. It may arise—as, for instance, in dorsal curvature—from diminished action, that is, from some cause diminishing respiration on the one side, or from increased function on the other. When these circumstances have caused the vertebræ to rotate, and the spine to curve, certain changes in the column are produced; and it will be desirable to examine what those are, and the signs which should lead us to consider them remediable or the reverse.

Firstly, to elucidate what these changes are, I must, even at the risk of repetition, refer to the explanation which I have given of the curves induced by the erect posture in the straight infantile spine, and to the fact that these

normal antero-posterior curves are permitted
by compression of the intervertebral substances, by tension and relaxation of opposed
ligaments. This being the case, it must like-
wise be the fact that the normal lateral bending and rotation, such as I have measured and
described, produce analogous compressions and
tension of different parts. And again, when
the lateral flexion and torsion begin to become
morbid and fixed, can it be for a moment supposed that other conditions in the column
itself, beyond those above mentioned, exist?
At first, then, a spine affected with lateral
curvature is by an extraneous force so placed
that the intervertebral substances are compressed, the ligaments relaxed on the concave
aspect, while on the convex face of the curve
a contrary disposition prevails. This is posi-
tively all;* the column itself is normal, but is
held in a certain posture by a force outside
itself. We have never, or hardly ever, a
chance in England of making a thorough
examination after death of a spine in the first

---

* Cases of rickety spine are here excluded.

stages of lateral curvature. By the word thorough I mean such an examination as can permit us to compare bony with ligamentous and muscular change. To make this investigation, the column, together with some portions of the ribs, must necessarily be removed, and the parts rigidly measured. There are, it is true, in the various pathological museums of London, sundry specimens of curved spine, but nearly all these are rickety cases, and the others that I have seen are old bones, certainly not under forty years of age, and in which, therefore, the distortion must have lasted thirty years at least. Nevertheless, had these cases undergone the sort of scrutiny above indicated, some further information than that afforded by the dry skeleton would have been obtained. Some information, namely, such as that afforded by M. Cruveilhier, who examined a case of old and considerable distortion by careful measurement.

The curve extended from the 3rd to the 11th dorsal vertebra, and was so severe that the radius measured 189 millimètres, the aggregate thickness of these 9 bones was on the

convex side 222, on the concave 125 millimètres. The fibrocartilages measured on the
convex side 65, on the other 45 millimètres.
That is to say, that even in so old a case the
bones had altered to only $\frac{1}{30}$ of their length,
the cartilaginous discs to $\frac{1}{4}$. Moreover, the
9th, 10th, and 11th bones of the back were
equally thick on their two sides, while on the
convex sides the intervertebral cartilages were
28, on the other only 16 millimètres in depth
(' *Bulletin de la Société Anatomique*, 1846.')
This, with another case also quoted by Mal-
gaigne, but from a journal to which I have no
access (' *Journal de Maisonabe* '), is conclusive
concerning the cartilaginous compression in
this disease. It must be recollected that these
measurements are taken from an old curve in
a dead recumbent subject, in which the flaccid
spine supports no weight, and on which the
vital resiliency of ligamentous parts has disappeared. They represent, therefore, with
regard to hard structures, the same difference;
but with regard to soft ones, a less difference
than during life.

Having thus proved that the bend and

torsion of a lateral curve is permitted by
compression and tension of ligamentous parts,
it becomes our duty to discover what amount,
and what duration of curve will have been
sufficient to deform these parts beyond their
power of recovery. I know of no direct
means whereby this question may be answered.
A belief expressed at the Royal Medical and
Chirurgical Society,* that all lateral curvatures accompanied by rotation are incurable,
affects only the choice of treatment. Nevertheless an indirect method of answering this
question by estimating the normal resiliency
of the intervertebral substance lies within our
reach.

Herr Hirschfeld, of Prague, the first to
doubt that the thickness of the vertebral bodies
varies with the direction of the normal curves,
goes further in his experiments. He cleared
from a spine all the muscles, leaving the ligaments intact; then, by cutting through all
the pedicles, separated the bodies. All the
normal curves disappeared, the intervertebral

* 'The Lancet,' Nov. 20th, 1865.

substances increasing their thickness behind
in the lumbar and cervical regions; in front
in the dorsal, and decreasing on the opposite
aspects.

I have not been able to discover the age of
the subject in the above description, and
therefore twice repeated for myself this
troublesome experiment: once on a subject
aged thirty-four; and again on one aged
forty-three. Precisely the same result followed, nor could I find any difference between
the two in the rapidity with which the spine
became straight. Thus although in these
cases the intervertebral cushions had been
subject to compression on one side, and
elongation on the other, during thirty-two
and forty-one years respectively (I deduct
two years for infancy previous to walking),
yet these substances retained all their elasticity. Therefore a lateral curve also must have
lasted a long time before those cushions lose
their power of recovery.

We now may go on to the next point. I
shall, when describing certain curative means,
have occasion to speak of the influence of the

recumbent posture in annulling or diminishing lateral curvature; for some amelioration, except in very severe cases, is always produced by the prone position. Abnormal curves of moderate amount entirely disappear, while those of greater amount and older date are only ameliorated, and the oldest, sharpest curves may not perhaps be straightened at all. The amount of benefit in this posture will, at all events, represent the amount of resiliency left in the ligamentous portions of the spine. In the first class this is altogether unimpaired, and if we can remove the extrinsic restraining force the column will straighten itself. In the next class the diminished elasticity of ligamentous matter is such, that we must, besides reinstating the impaired muscular balance, apply certain force to supplement for a time the lost resiliency. In the third and more restricted class, all that we can do is to prevent the case getting worse—to relieve pain from pressure in abnormal directions, and in some few to obtain a certain, though probably a small, amount of improvement in form.

CHAPTER VI.

PRINCIPLES OF TREATMENT.

ANY person pointing out a better method of treating some disease, is bound to show wherein the old one is defective; and it therefore devolves upon me to demonstrate the theoretical and practical errors of the prevalent mode of treating lateral curvature. But if I state that by exclusive and special dealing with this disease its treatment has got into a vicious groove—if I direct attention, however strongly, to some of the points in orthopædic practice, which appear to me faulty and injurious—it must be permitted me once for all to say, that no personal ill-will whatever guides my pen. However badly I may think of this practice, and of the mode in which it is carried out, I entertain no other feeling than of all due professional respect towards those gentlemen who practise a system from which I am conscientiously bound to differ.

The multitudinous theoretical errors, which have attributed the origin of lateral curvature to sundry causes already discussed, have naturally led to corresponding misdirection of treatment. This misdirection has in all its forms much the same tendency, since, whatever be the theory of causes, the proximate defect has always been attributed to the spinal bones, ligaments, or muscles, and the treatment, therefore, has been aimed at those organs. So exhaustive have been the devices employed, that if these were really the peccant parts, they must inevitably have yielded to some one or more of the vast powers brought to bear upon their evil influence. Sometimes, with the idea that these organs are too weak to support the body's weight, patients have been kept on their backs for years, the head and trunk have been upheld in slings and cages, they have been exercised by gymnastic performances. Sometimes supposed too strong, the muscles have been cut, or again stretched

by machines formed and used like gallows;
also on couches—some of which act longitu-
dinally, others by endeavouring to bend the
back contrary to the curve. These devices,
many of which are equally ingenious and com-
plicated, possess every requisite for success,
save any influence on the deforming cause;
we therefore find that they have fallen into
complete desuetude, except certain exercises
occasionally employed, but still misdirected to
the spinal muscles, and the use of certain
machinery. Indeed, at the present time the
treatment of this deformity is almost or entirely limited to the application, screwing and
unscrewing of a mechanism termed a spinal
support, which therefore requires some description before we proceed to consider its
value or the reverse.

The instrument referred to is represented
in the annexed figure, borrowed from an orthopædic work published a year or two ago.
Its foundation consists of a steel band passing
round the hips and abdomen, which carries
two steel rods provided with crutch-handles,
and also two movable levers bearing plates

of the same metal, that are to be placed on
each side over the ribs. The object aimed at
is this :— The patient
is to be placed in
the machine; the
steel belt is fastened
around the abdomen ;
the shoulders are
strapped to the
crutch handles; then,
by a simple mechan-
ism, these are length-

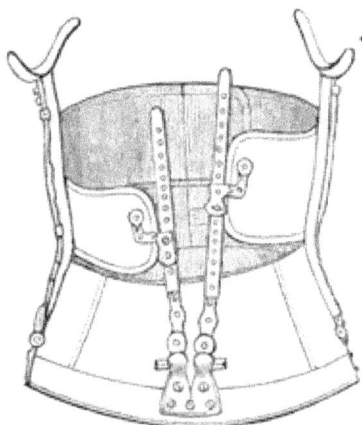

A "Spinal Support."

ened so as to lift the shoulders, with the
intention of extending the spine; further-
more, the movable levers are screwed so as to
force the plates with a certain pressure against
the protuberant parts of the ribs and loins.

The rounded parts about hip and buttocks
alone afford, however, no sufficient means of
fixing a band immovably, and unless the steel
circle from which all these levers act be immovable or nearly so, the force of the screws,
&c., will twist and displace the belt, but cannot
affect the spine. To gain the necessary im-
mobilisation, therefore, sundry swathings and

bandages must be added. One of these sur-
mounts the metallic pelvic band, and, enclosing
the loins, is tightly laced over the abdomen;
while others, passing forward from the crutch-
handled staves, are similarly fastened in front
of the chest. This scaffolding aims at placing
the individual in entire immobility as far as
the trunk is concerned; any sideways movement, any bending forwards or backwards,
any turning round, are to be rendered impossible; the figure must move all in one
piece, like a Dutch doll. This, I say, is the
object aimed at, and which, if the instrument
is to have influence on the spine, must be
attained; fortunately, however, for the well-
being of the patients it is pretty nearly impossible to arrive at this end, as any one who
has endeavoured to hold the trunk even of a
baby still, is aware. Thus the immense
power and flexibility of the figure soon causes
this or that steel rod to yield in one or the
other direction, giving the body sufficient
liberty to make life endurable, and to negative
the supposed influence of the levers on the
spine. The instrument then simply resem-

bles heavy stays of an exceptionally un-
wholesome construction.

For there is another portion of this machinery which does not yield : the tight swathings above described, although they may slip
up or down enough to let the scaffolding
rods give, encircle the abdomen and effectually
check its respiratory movements. But we
have already seen (p. 39) that anything
which by preventing the breathing movements of the belly, forces that function to be
unduly pectoral, is in itself an efficient cause
of dorsal curvature.

The instrument therefore absolutely increases the root of the evil, not only by the
abdominal constriction, but by the belt over
the chest, which presses back the ribs chiefly,
of course, on the side of the largest lung—the
right. Such confinement and such compression of important organs have their natural
effect, and few girls emerge from such treatment without considerable loss of health ; and
in cases where even slight predisposition exists,
consumption is induced, as many physicians
in London are aware. Nevertheless, I must

in justice say that in a certain very small percentage of cases these mechanisms have effected some good. Such cases belong to the class of weight-bearing curves, and they have been benefited by relieving the spine of the weight of that shoulder which lies on its convex side. Such object can, however, be effected by a far simpler method, which does not imprison the trunk at all, as I shall hereafter show.

Lest it be imagined that I am unjust towards this mechanism in asserting that it benefits only a very small percentage of cases, and lest my testimony concerning an instrument which I never use be considered valueless, I will here sum up shortly the experience of those who do use them, and who would certainly be disposed to give the most favourable view of their value. Dr. Little says : *—" They are not adapted to the removal of the primary causes of lateral curvature ; they cannot, therefore, be employed as curative means." And, in a very recent work,†—" Notwith-

---

* 'On Deformities of the Human Spine,' p. 379.
† 'On Spinal Weakness and Spinal Curvature,' p. 65.

standing all that has been said or written in relation to lateral curvature and spinal supports, no spinal apparatus or support hitherto designed is able to overcome rotation of the spine." Mr. Tamplin and Mr. Brodhurst both eulogise these scaffoldings; but it is difficult to find what results they gain, or expect to gain, from their use. Mr. Adams, whose treatise on the subject is more exhaustive, says:*—"I have no hesitation in expressing my conviction that if these cases be submitted to treatment before any very obvious external deformity has occurred, they are generally curable within one or two years. In some instances, especially if an hereditary tendency to spinal curvature exist, and the girl is of feeble constitutional power, a longer period may be required." Which appears to mean that if a strong young girl of healthy parentage be fastened up in one of these machines for two years, she may be cured in that period of a deformity which can hardly be said to exist. A further insight is afforded

---

* 'Lectures on Curvature of the Spine,' p. 326.

by the expressions of two of the above-named
gentlemen at the Royal Medical and Chirurgical Society meeting of January 9th, 1866 :*
—"The result of my experience has been to
convince me that where lateral curvature
existed in any marked degree, and before
it amounted to an external deformity, it
is essentially an incurable affection" (Mr.
Adams). "When rotation has taken place"
(the *primum mobile* of the deviation), "appliances are useless." The causes of so sad an
experience require some comment. A malady
may be non-amenable to treatment, from posi-
tive incurability, or from impropriety of
measures taken. Now, firstly, it would be
very unwise to conclude that a malady is
incurable if a certain application had done no
good, but probably some harm. Secondly, it
seems *primâ facie* absurd to affirm that a slight
deviation of form in a young person is incurable. Thirdly, the result of my experience leads to a very different conclusion.

Another device, spinal myotomy—already

---

* Vide 'The Lancet' of Jan. 23rd, 1866.

justly condemned and dead,—will here require
no further notice or mention at my hands.

The plan of treatment which I have pursued
for some years, and which I am about to describe, differs from the prevalent method of
Orthopædy in several very essential principles.
The latter, by preventing normal breathing,
adds to the causes of deformity, and it im-
mobilizes the trunk as far as it possibly can,
thus debilitating the spinal muscles, which,
after all, must uphold the column. The former
is adapted to strengthen the weakened muscles, to prevent undue pectoral breathing,
or, at least, to obviate its injurious effects.
Thus, for both forms of curvature described
in foregoing chapters, the treatment resolves
itself into three portions—viz., support, position, and exercise. The two last divisions
might strictly be classified together, since
every remedial position, necessitating activity
of certain muscles, is in truth an exercise;
nevertheless, it will be more convenient for
our purpose to retain the classification as
above, premising only that by position I mean
the ordinance of a certain immoving pos-

ture; by exercise certain movements are denoted.

Regarding supports, which must be of different forms in varying cases, it will be desirable to say a few words which apply to them all. In the first place, they must never be rigid: to fix immovably for an indefinite time a portion of the body, which is intended by nature to be mobile, at first weakens and subsequently destroys muscular power—that power, namely, on which we must rely, at the end of treatment, for the maintenance of an erect posture. In the next place, the direction in which the force is to act must be considered; and, to do this fairly, I must again revert to the change produced in a lateral curve by recumbency. In my earlier studies of lateral curvature I was much struck by the fact, that in commencing cases the curve vanishes when the patient lies down. In a later stage the curvature, though greatly diminishing, does not entirely disappear. I tried, therefore, in these latter cases, to increase the effect of posture by longitudinal traction. Instantly the curves were aggra-

vated : no matter how gradual or how sudden
was the force employed, it always increased
the curves according to its amount. I then
tried the same expedient in cases in which the
morbid posture was entirely annulled by position ; and in these, when traction was made,
the curve reappeared. This was equally the
case, whether the upward or counter-extension
was made from the head and neck, or from the
shoulders and upper part of the chest. I then
perceived this fact,—that recumbency, while it
obviates the lateral bend, does not affect rotation ; or, to make this phrase easier, by ex-
pansion, I would say :—On a rotated spine the
erectores spinæ act in a lateral direction (since
they turn with the bones), and bend the column sideways. In the erect posture those
muscles are in full action, and the deviation,
therefore, well marked. In the prone position the organs are at rest, and the lateral
curve ceases : rotation, however, being dependent on other causes, still continues. All
muscles, however, are excited by stretching ;
so, when in recumbency traction is employed,
the erectors contract and reproduce the curve.

Hence, to use force in the longitudinal direction, with the hope of straightening the spine, is a physiological and mechanical blunder.

Let us return to the curves which only partially disappear during recumbency. Force upwards and downwards—i. e., in the direction of the crutch-handles in orthopædic instruments, aggravates the curve; but the effect of force at right angles to the spine is quite different : no muscular effort is excited thereby,—hence very little power, save in old cases, will straighten the column. Indeed, when a patient with curvature stands before the surgeon, he instinctively places a hand on each side at the greatest point of deviation, and, by pressing in opposite directions, finds that, according to the severity of the case, he can entirely or partially restore the straight line of the spine. The bandage which I use is contrived simply to render permanent, by an elastic force, the office which the surgeon's hands can only temporarily fulfil.

With regard to the other two items of treatment, I would only remark that, to devise exercise for any deformity, the origin-

ator will act upon his views of the causes of
disease, and of the actions which he thinks
most calculated to obviate them. In following
out this sort of work, he finds certain methods
fail to call forth the power he intended, or
they may not only act as he calculated, but
evoke also other and unexpected forces, which
subvert the object in view, so that modifica-
tion or abandonment of some cherished design
becomes necessary. The actions and powers
of a machine are easily reckoned—a certain
force, a given number, and size of cogs or
levers, and the result is certain; but nothing
is more subtle or varied than the acts of the
human body. I have found not unfrequently
that a position maintained by certain muscles
will, after a time, when fatigue has come on
suddenly, leave those parts at rest, and with
an almost imperceptible change of posture,
will employ for a short period another, or
rather a number of other sets. So also, in
different persons, there is some appreciable
but indescribable difference in the mode of
muscular action, so that the one is best fitted
by exercise or posture in a certain position,

another requires some slight variation. But
in all this part of my method, as well as in
the construction of the bandage, it has been
my desire to make the treatment " direct."
The most important postures which I shall
describe, the respiratory and lumbar exercises,
the bandage and arm support, are calculated
on that principle. They are aimed straight at
the mark they are intended to hit, and in my
experience the shafts fly true ; yet, before
describing the detail of my method, it will be
well to mention an example of what I mean
by the term " directness of treatment," only
premising that no established curve can be so
easily cured ; the case simply illustrates the
advantages of an attack upon the cause of
curvature.

Miss A. W——, aged nineteen, had long been the
subject of strumous inflammation of the left knee,
which occasionally had brought her under the threat
of amputation. When I saw her in January, 1861, the
swollen joint was discharging by three sinuses, from
which small particles of bone had frequently come. In
eighteen months she was able to walk with the aid of
a stick. After an interval of two years, on seeing her
again, I observed that the lumbar spine was crooked,
though she wore a thicker boot on the left foot. This

curve continued while she sat on a level seat, and only partially disappeared when she lay down. Seeing that she walked and stood a great deal, and that the obliquity of the pelvis caused the spinal curve, I wished to counteract this effect by placing her while sitting in such a position as should reverse this obliquity. I carefully measured the difference in length between the two limbs, and caused a cushion to be made of such wedge-shaped form as should, when she sat upon it, lift the right side of the pelvis to the same extent as it was depressed in standing. This, of course, reversed the pelvic obliquity, and in time caused the spine to curve while she was seated in the contrary direction. This means and a bandage, to be hereafter described, sufficed to annul the lateral curvature.

CHAPTER VII.

TREATMENT OF LUMBAR CURVE.

In stating, at the end of the last chapter, that a spinal curvature cannot be cured simply by making a patient sit for some time on a sloping seat, it was, in fact, merely asserted that this, like other diseases, must be treated with reference to its severity and cause. For this reason, much pains has been taken to define the essential causality of each class of curvature; and it must be permitted me here to recall these facts, that while each class of primary dorsal curvature is always followed by a lumbar curve, so a curve primarily lumbar calls forth a dorsal arc in the contrary direction,—the bend thus produced by the primary one being in each case called secondary or compensating. In all these maladies it is desirable to obtain the earliest symptoms indicative of the disease ; and I would remind the reader that in lumbar curvature a peculiar backward projection of one side of the pelvis is earlier than its lateral projection—earlier also than lateral deviation; but contemporary, or only slightly preceding, an amount of rotation which the practised hand can detect.

This prominence marks the causality of the disease which we have traced to some changed posture of pelvis and thighs. The direct and natural plan of treatment will therefore most evidently be to correct these faulty conditions ; and no doubt, if we could always encounter the malady in its earliest stages, such treatment would in itself prove efficacious, as in the case related in the previous chapter. The fact is, however, that the distortion rarely comes under skilled observation in the earlier part of its course ; and thus we have to encounter, besides mere habit and the influence of superincumbent weight, passive shortening of certain muscles, debility of others, and, in tolerably advanced cases, contraction of ligaments. Sufficient and commensurate treatment for an established curve will naturally include the divisions of treatment already discussed, which are destined to counteract those different defects.

Firstly, it is of the utmost importance to place the patient at ease; and while conversing, or asking questions concerning health or age, &c., to watch the posture assumed, to observe the position of the feet, or the mode of sitting, whether cross-legged on one side, &c., to get at the habits and occupations, and to conclude, as far as possible, what circumstances in the daily life have given rise to that posture of the lower parts of the body which may have called forth the deformity. Although these may sometimes escape investigation, yet careful study will very frequently lead to the detection of the injurious habit, and this, of course, must be at once attacked.

Our first curative means, namely position,* is represented chiefly by the sloping seat—a device for lifting that side of the pelvis which is abnormally depressed, whose action may be

---

* It may be as well to repeat that all remedial position implies to a considerable extent exercise of those muscles which in the malposture are unused.

thus explained. The accompanying engraving is taken from one of my patients who had

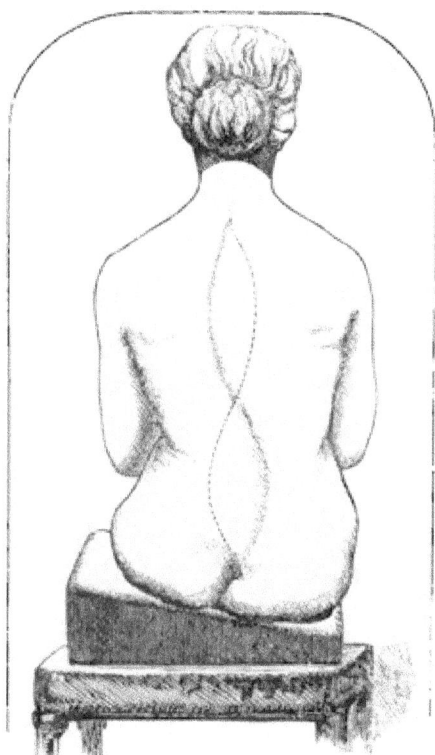

The Sloping Seat.

all but recovered from a rather severe lumbar
curve, represented by the dotted line. The
figure is placed upon a seat, which slopes from
left to right, *i. e.*, from the convex to the concave side ; and it is from this figure evident
that, if we artificially lift the part of the

pelvis which lies to the convex side, the spine,
forced by the law of balance, will tend to
assume a curve in the contrary direction.
The reader also will aid his comprehension of
this condition if he will look back to p. 50, at
the diagram which represents the undulations
of the column in a figure rocking from side to
side. The block in the above engraving upon
which the torso is seated hardly represents,
however, the mechanism by which I work in
these cases. I have a stool with a top, which,
lying horizontal, can be raised at one end, by
means of a winch and cogged wheels, so
gradually that the changes in the position of
the spine and the action of the muscles can,
during the elevation, be accurately observed.
Now, when the patient sits on this stool, with
the feet stretched out in front so that they do
not influence the trunk, and when the end on
the convex side is slowly lifted, one observes
the following changes :—firstly, and previous
to any perceptible change in the lateral bend,
the lumbar vertebræ begin to relinquish their
torsion, to untwist themselves; the parts on
the convex side become less hard, those on the

concave more so, and the transverse processes
sink deeper—are not so evident; the lateral
inflexion then also becomes affected, and in all
but severe cases it will disappear at the same
time that the torsion ceases. I have, however,
in a previous sentence, used the phrase, "the
spine *tends* to assume a contrary curve,"
because I would guard against any appearance of exaggeration; therefore I must not be
supposed to say that an established lumbar
curve can be at once inverted by such means,
or even that it will be immediately effaced.
An evident and manifest improvement is,
however, while the figure is sitting, instantly
produced, and as the back becomes stronger,
the patient can use the device for longer
periods, so as to keep the spine in a more
normal, and at last, with the assistance of
other means, in a perfectly normal position
during the greater part of the day.

Simple as the device appears, its efficacy is
very considerable; indeed although, when I
first began to employ this mechanism on de-
formed patients, there were many reasons to
expect very considerable advantage from its

use, I was not prepared for the amount of
change induced : nevertheless its regulation
requires considerable care ; indeed, there are
few things in practice more difficult than to
fix the degree of slope, and the time of
employment which will be beneficial.

By means of the contrivance for regulating
the angle of inclination without obliging the
patient to rise or use any unnecessary muscular effort, one can, however, arrive at a
very accurate judgment of the amount of force
expended on the spine, and the action of the
lumbar muscles during the elevation of one
side must be carefully watched ; I would also
point out that it is partly the diminishing
torsion in the lumbar, the primary curve,
and partly the behaviour of the dorsal
(secondary) curvature, which must serve as
an index.   The secondary curve is thus available, because since it is consecutive it is also
less indelible, and because the longer sweep
of the arc renders such change more appreciable.   While we bear in mind that a slight
degree of slope will produce little or no
benefit, a violent inclination, or too long

a period of use, may be productive of very considerable evil.

Emma T——, aged seventeen years and a half, came to me on Feb. 16th, 1863. She is employed at a sewing machine, which she always drives with the right foot : is strongly built, but now pale, and evidently out of health, suffering from profuse leucorrhœa. On examining the back I found a considerable primary lumbar curve to the right, with a secondary dorsal curvature, both of which only partially disappeared on lying down. Seeing the depressed state of health, I only ordered tonics, with similar regimen, and certain recommendations about the mode of working.

March 2nd.—Better. Finds great difficulty in working with the left foot, and it is often impossible to do so. I ordered a sloping seat, being very careful to fix both the angle and the time of use small, on account of state of health; also ordered a bandage as hereafter described.

April 2nd.—Up to the middle of the month considerable improvement had taken place, and I had simply advised continuation of the same course. At the above date, however, she was looking very ill, and complained of severe pains in the back and loins. I found that her cousin, seeing the improvement produced by gentle means, had counselled her to have the slope made higher (nearly doubled) and to use it the chief part of the day. On examination, I found the back less well ; the muscles on the right of the spine were swollen and tender to the touch ; the loins so weak that she could with difficulty sit or stand upright.

I

She was ordered to leave off the sloping seat; the
bandage was tightened; and the cousin was shown
how to rub the muscles upwards with a liniment of
ammonia, chloroform, and opium.

May 7th.—As the patient had now quite recovered
from the pain and weakness, the use of the sloping seat
was cautiously resumed; and from this time the case
went on uninterruptedly till I discharged her from
care, quite straight, on Dec. 16th, 1863.

Such device can, from its very nature, only
be used while sitting; hence, when the back
becomes more straight, and the lumbar muscles
on the concave side sufficiently strong, we
may carry on the same principle in the
standing posture by ordering an additional
sole of cork to one boot, *i. e.*, that on the convex
side of the curve. For the first day or two
the patient finds this awkward, but very soon
becomes accustomed to it. Nevertheless, I
only use it in severe cases, and for those
patients whose power is good and health
confirmed.

Exercise is in a great measure included in
the position enforced by the sloping seat and
the high shoe; but we may advantageously
add to these certain calisthenics destined more
especially to increase the power of the muscles

at the lower part of the spine, on the concave side of the spine. Space forbids my entering very fully into details ; I will simply mention those which I have found most advantageous. Let the lumbar curve be to the left : the patient, with both knees perfectly straight, stands on a block or book from one to three inches high, as the case may demand, and with the right foot so close to the edge of the block that, by just separating the limbs, the sole passes over the border. Still keeping the knees quite straight, the right foot is by action at the hips made to sink till its sole rests fairly on the ground for a short period, both knees being kept straight ; then it is replaced on the book, and this manœuvre is repeated for a prescribed time, and at a certain rate. A chair is placed against the wall, the patient standing sideways to the wall, balances herself with the left hand upon it, and planting the left foot on the chair, slowly lifts herself until she stands upright. Standing with her back to the wall, the patient slowly lifts the left knee forward till the thigh is at right angles to the body, and gradually lets the limb fall

again, repeating this movement slowly and
rhythmically. After a time the foot is to be
weighted according to the strength of the
patient.

An exercise very valuable in long-standing
and severe cases, for stretching ligaments on
the concave side of the spine, is the following. The patient stands with the back to
the wall, and, if possible, with the left side
against the-corner wall, or some upright piece
of furniture, as a piano or bookcase, so that
she may be sure of not deviating from the
perpendicular to that side. A block, of care-
fully-proportioned thickness, is placed under
the right foot. Fixing the right arm a-kimbo,
she quickly and forcibly (according to her
strength) bends the upper part of the body
sideways to the right, and repeats this several
times. The back must be kept against the
wall, the knees kept rigidly straight, and if
the limbs be rather weak, or the patient
awkward, a napkin or round towel passed
round the hips, and secured to the wall on
her left, must uphold the due position of the
pelvis.

These are the more important among the exercises which I employ. They are to be used with great caution, and from time to time the surgeon must watch them, lest any awkward trick in their performance render them useless or injurious.

It is necessary to warn the reader against ordering any of these exercises, indeed any part of the treatment, lightly or incautiously. Simple as they may seem—indeed are,—they are also *direct*, and as a force applied directly is the more potent in proportion to this quality, so, if improperly employed, its power for evil will be great.

The form of support which I use in this description of curve is founded on the principle of using force as nearly as possible in the direction of the radii of the curves. The annexed figure shows a lumbar curve to the right, together with the simplest form of bandage. A round well-covered strap, about the size of the little finger, passing round the upper part of the thigh, supports on the hip a triangular pad strapped to the part; from the two upper angles a well-fitting piece of some strong material passes round the loins. This portion becomes broader, so that its greatest breadth is over the most prominent part of the curve; from that point as it passes round in front it tapers again. In the view as given, no fastening or other contrivance is visible, but in front the band is rendered elastic by the insertion of a strong india-rubber ring, and here, too, is added a means of fastening, as well as an arrangement whereby the surgeon can himself fix and vary the degree of tension without leaving it to the hap-hazard will of the patient. The object of keeping all the elastic force in front is this, that, while it perfectly allows all desirable movements of the body, the power supporting and upholding the lumbar curvature acts from right to left, and aids in obviating the morbid torsion of vertebræ in the contrary direction. However, when the curvature is extreme, or where, as happens in rare cases, torsion is not commensurate with the lateral curve, I insert elastic power behind also. If the secondary curve be well marked, and does not disappear when the patient lies

down, if the patient be muscularly weak, or if
the part of the bandage just described have a

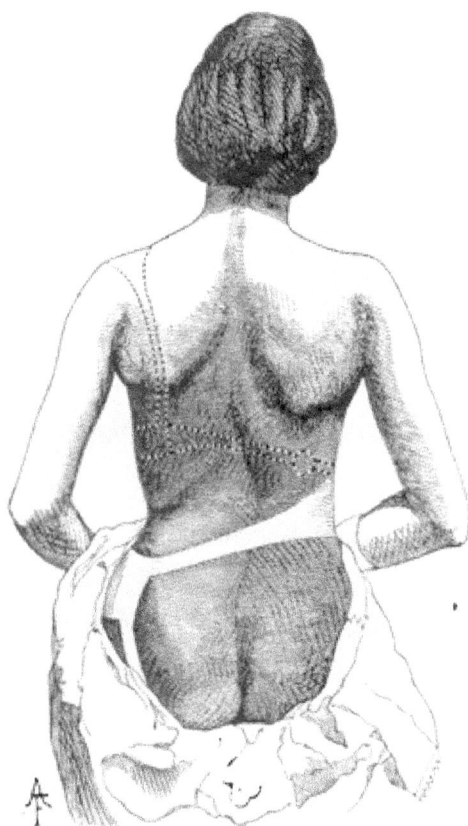

The simplest form of support is marked in white, the additional
portion (generally required) by dotted lines.

tendency to slip, the other portion (marked in
dotted lines) must be added. This simply
consists of a band (supplied with the same

elastic force and means of securing the proper tension) passing to a pad opposite the most prominent part of the dorsal curve, and supplied with a shoulder-strap to avoid slipping. The mode in which this latter part is arranged varies in different cases, according to the slope of the shoulders, position and size of mammæ, &c.

The advantages which such support possesses over steel instruments are, lightness, the absence of absolute restraint, and the direction of the force being transverse to the chord of curve. The round form of the band at the top of the thigh prevents any cutting, and the fact that the force is exerted upon it at right angles to its direction causes the tension on that part to be very slight.

These broad principles must suffice as the guides of treatment. One exercise will be found most applicable in one case, while another may be found suitable to a different patient, and what is advisable in one stage is not useful in another. I do not know that I can give any certain guide to choice; and, although a considerable experience enables me now to judge what will be most available, I always let the movement be performed in my presence, under careful supervision. It is, however, well always to prescribe the less powerful exercises for weak persons, and in the weakest to leave all muscular exertion out of the question, and work by position and support alone. The advantage of this plan will be seen in some of the cases detailed.

As a matter of prognosis it is well to be aware that the curves primarily lumbar are more obstinate, *i. e.*, require a longer time for cure than the same amount of dorsal curvature; but that unless far advanced, and especially if evil habits of position and wrong modes of taking exercise be avoided, they belong essentially to the category of curable disease.

Miss E. C., aged 22, came to me May 5th, 1866, with a well marked spinal curve, which was only suspected, however, a few weeks ago. She now suffers considerable pain in the lower part of the left chest and lumbar region; for this she underwent treatment directed to the digestive organs, and thinks that she was much weakened thereby. During the last year her health has failed; she has dysmenorrhœa, faulty appetite, and sleeps badly; is pale and exsanguineous.

I found that there was considerable spinal deviation, with retrocession of and lateral projection of the back part of the pelvis; a compensating curve had formed in the dorsal region. A plumb-line, dropped from 7th cervical vertebra, crossed the S-shaped curve between the 9th and 10th dorsal vertebræ; the 2nd lumbar spinous process lay 1 inch four lines to the left of this line, the 5th dorsal $\frac{3}{4}$ inch to the right. The left transverse processes of the loins formed easily-felt prominences, while a hollow lay on the right side of the loins. The patient being so far out of health, it seemed to me desirable to proceed very gently; I therefore simply ordered her to sit on a seat sloping $1\frac{1}{2}$ inch in the foot, for a quarter of an hour twice a day, and after this to repose on the couch for an equal space. Tonics of steel and some aloes were prescribed.

May 14th.—There is a certain small improvement; a support, such as described in the text, was adapted, at but a small degree of tension.

June 1st.—At a previous visit the tension of the bandage was increased, and the use of the seat ordered for thrice in the day. Her health is now better; she has all but lost the pains complained of, and the complexion is less bloodless; appetite is also improved.

June 28th.—The health has manifestly improved. The curvature now has the following measurements:— 2nd lumbar 1 inch, 5th dorsal $\frac{1}{2}$ inch from mesial line. —To continue with a rather tighter bandage.

July 14th.—The back continues to improve, and the

patient has gained strength considerably.—Ordered to have a boot ⅓ inch higher on the left than on the right side.

Sept. 10th.—The patient, seen occasionally during the interval, has continued with these ordonnances; has greatly improved, so much so that the straight line of silk between 7th cervical vertebra and middle of sacrum lies over all the spinous processes—but in the loins they only skirt the right side, in the back the left side of those projections. Rotation is still marked enough to enable one just to feel the left lumbar transverse process. The lady considers herself well, and it is only my insistance which causes her to continue under treatment.

Dec. 17th.—I now also consider this patient well, since I can detect no lateral deviation, no sign of rotation, and the parts are equally hard on both sides of the spine. She also can turn her body equally to both sides, as shewn by the rotation measurer.

June 10th, 1867.—This patient wished to see me again previous to a projected marriage; I examined the back, and still found no deviation whatever.

Alice B——, a short, but strongly built and muscular girl, aged 17, was brought to me with a sharp and well-defined lumbar curve to the right, Nov., 1865.

The backward projection of the right sacro-iliac joint was particularly well marked—the rotation at the loins strong, while the curve itself was sharper and more defined than usual. On watching the positions which the patient assumed, I found that she, in walking and standing, turned the right knee and foot a

good deal in; and on a subsequent visit, as I gave her
some portion of bandage to stitch, I observed that as
she sat to work she threw the left leg well across the
right, and leaned her left elbow on the thigh of that
side. She was a shoe-binder, and worked in this attitude a good number of hours daily.

I explained the absolute necessity of changing this
posture; ordered a sloping seat, highest on the right
side, to be used only a short time, thrice in the day,
namely, at meals. By degrees the time of its use was
increased, until she was able to work upon it while
sitting, and very shortly after a strong lumbar bandage
was employed.

This case improved rapidly in the first two months
of treatment, during the greater part of which she had
discontinued her employment. After that interval,
and during a period of three months, the progress
became slower, and she lost health to a certain degree.
I took her into hospital, April, 1866, and had her exercises and the posture of sitting properly superintended.
I also had her right boot heightened by a piece of cork
half an inch thick.

July 30th, 1866.—The case had now very much improved, and as another employment —domestic service —
has been found for the girl, I have dismissed her from
the hospital; in the mean time she has been cured of
her awkward tricks of sitting and walking, and the
back, while the bandage is *in situ*, is not far from
straight.

Oct. 5th.—This patient has been seen about every
fortnight, and the back has been improving. Occasionally a certain amount of the cork has been cut from

the sole, and for the last three weeks the boots have been of equal thickness.

The back is now quite straight, the girl stands well upright on the two feet, and the parts on each side of the spinous processes are equally hard and protuberant.

Miss L——, aged 24, has for some time been suffering from a curvature of the spine, and has worn for more than four years the usual form of orthopædic support. She came to me on the 5th May, 1866, and gave the following history.

About five years ago, she, being previously well and hearty, began to lose health, and suffered pain in the back; these symptoms increased, menstruation became irregular, and all but ceased; appetite failed, breathing became short and difficult. She was taken to a practitioner near her residence, and he, in examining her, found signs of curvature, and sent her to London in 1861. The gentleman whom she consulted told her that she must remain some considerable time in town, and wear an iron support. She did remain the greater part of a year in London; during which time the instrument was screwed up, at first thrice, then twice a week, and afterwards once a week. At the end of rather more than ten months she found herself unable to stay longer, or to afford further treatment. The instrument was very much tightened, so as to last longer without alteration, and she left London. At that time she was suffering more pain in the back; her health was much broken, and she was, when the instrument was removed, more crooked, although she says that when the scaffolding was tightly screwed she was a little taller. She had, however, lost health more rapidly; had become very thin; was very easily wearied; scarcely able to walk; her appetite was very small, and somewhat capricious; she suffered also considerable pain, chiefly on the right side. She continued to wear the instrument for some time, in the country; but after a little more than two months her strength so failed that she was obliged to take almost entirely to bed and the sofa, leaving off the scaffolding. Her health now began to improve again, and as she shortly was enabled to get about, she became again desirous of improving the shape of the spine, and resumed the support, but found again that her health failed, and was obliged to discontinue it. After six weeks more she consulted me.

At the date above given, I found her pale and weak; she could not sit up for more than a few minutes at a time; appetite bad and capricious; pulse small; menstruation irregular and scanty.

The following measurements give the curvature of the spine. A silk thread between the 7th cervical vertebra and the middle of the sacrum crossed exactly over the 9th dorsal spinous process. The second lumbar spine was $1\frac{1}{2}$ inch to the right, the 5th dorsal was $\frac{5}{8}$ inch to the left. When she lay down the curve decreased.

In this case it was, I felt, necessary to be very cautious in the application of any treatment. I ordered therefore at first a seat, sloping only $1\frac{1}{2}$ inch in 15, for ten minutes twice in the day, and to rest on the back immediately afterwards, and to take steel wine twice a day—a steel and aloes pill night and morning.

May 18th —She is better in health ; the back has, of course, hardly altered, but the hardness and protuberance of parts on the right of the spine are rather less marked. A bandage has been constructed, and this was now applied with but little tension; to continue the sloping seat.

June 12th.—The health has decidedly improved, and the patient has gained flesh with rather remarkable rapidity : the back also is better, the improvement being chiefly manifest by the decreasing rotation, as seen in the greater equality of hardness on each side of the spine.

July 20th.—In the three or four visits since the former date there has only been to observe the gradual improvement in health and in the form of the back : a higher slope to the seat was instituted a fortnight ago ; the tension of the bandage has been two or three times re-arranged. The deviation was to-day carefully measured : 2nd lumbar spine $\frac{6}{8}$ inch to right, 5th dorsal $\frac{1}{4}$ to left. We have then gained $\frac{3}{8}$ on the lumbar (primary) curve, $\frac{1}{2}$ inch on the dorsal secondary curve. This, I may remark, is not uncommonly the case ; the secondary curve yields first and most.

August 28th.—Again I leave an interval in which there is nothing especial to remark ; improvement during that time has been however more rapid. Health is now very good. Menstruation has occurred with perfect regularity in the last three periods. She has sufficient colour and plumpness ; appetite good. Measurement gives the following result :—the 2nd lumbar spine lies so that the straight line is $\frac{1}{4}$ inch from its left border, and touches the right edge of the 5th dorsal vertebra.

Oct. 2nd.—The patient may now be considered well. The line of silk touches all the vertebræ; no transverse processes can be felt, but the parts on each side are equal in hardness and resiliency.

CHAPTER VIII.

ON THE TREATMENT OF DORSAL CURVATURE.

THE curvatures primarily dorsal form the
larger, the more important class of this deformity; and, before considering their treatment, I must beg leave to remind the reader
that in these forms of distortion torsion is the
first step, and that this is produced by preponderance of one serratus magnus over the
other. At this point the subject divides itself
into two; the preponderance is produced
either by overweighting one arm or by
excessively pectoral breathing, which chiefly
affects the side of the largest lung, namely,
the right.

Since, then, it is an essential part of the
principles advocated in this as in other of my
works, to determine the causes in each case,
and to treat the malady in accordance with
such cause, it is evident that in both classes

K

of the disease we must proceed by making the muscle on the convex side act less, that on the concave more; but since in each division the sort of work is different, so must the means taken to regulate its amount vary.

Let us first take the class of dorsal deformity originating in weight-bearing. These cases are chiefly met with among the working classes, and hence some difficulty in enforcing those alterations of habits and that attention to directions necessary for recovery. Nevertheless, much can be effected; and I have succeeded in curing many cases occurring in careful, well-conducted families, of this order. In the first place, it is necessary either to relieve the patient of the work, which produced the distortion, or to alter the mode of its performance. This work is generally carrying an infant or other burden : even long-continued sewing will produce slight curvature.* However we may wish to

---

* The mere movement of arm and forearm has, of course, nothing to do with the production of curvature. In all manipulations requiring evenness and uniformity of action, some part is kept fixed as a *point d'appui*. Those who have watched women at the needle

alter the mode of carrying burdens, it does not answer, save in the earliest stages, merely to tell a girl to use the other hand. I have, indeed, seen curves already well marked rendered worse by such ready and rather rough expedient. It is certainly best of all that the work cease for a time ; next best, that the burden be supported on each hand alternately. It is not at the moment when all the body is braced to perform some act of strength that the mischief is done, but in the longer lapse of duller work, when the antagonist muscles, or those that fix the points of

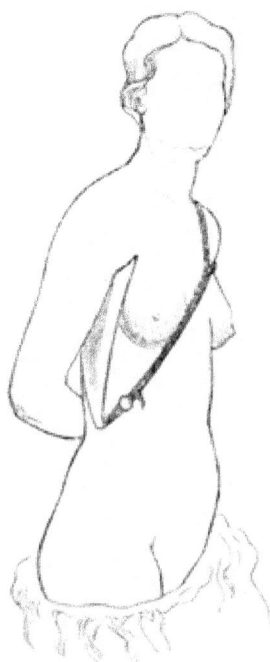

The Shoulder-sling for weight-bearing curves in early stage. The triangular part under the arm consists of a support whose upper side is elastic and soft. The belt portion is rendered elastic by the insertion of strong India-rubber rings.

will have observed that while the arm and forearm are allowed free play, the shoulder and blade-bone are held peculiarly still: this fixity, being produced almost entirely by the serratus, has its effect on the spine.

K 2

origin, neglect their duty, and allow the working muscles to lean upon bones and ligaments
for their support. We have, then, to obviate
the effects of constant or frequent pressure,
rather than of exceptional action ; and for this
reason I have devised a bandage, or sling, intended, not to support any great burden, but
simply to hang the weight of the right shoulder
on the left one (supposing curvature to the
right). The difficulty here is the fact of both
parts being on the same level. This was overcome by forming a strut, or beam, consisting of
a V-shaped piece of very thin, highly-tempered
steel, the upper ends of which are connected
by a thick india-rubber cord, upon which
(properly padded) the shoulder rests. From
the lower part of the point of the V sufficiently broad pieces of webbing pass behind
and in front of the body to the left shoulder,
and these bands are interrupted at intervals
by elastic cords disposed as rings, and by
buckles, with means of procuring proper tension. The bandage, properly managed, does
not cut. It fully answers its purpose of
relieving the right serratus ; but since, in all

but the earlier stages, it is necessary to produce also another effect, this sling is to be
combined generally with a support which I
have termed the "oblique bandage." The
object of this latter band is to uphold the
sides of the chest and spine; but, as it will
be described immediately, I will now merely
mention it as a band also to be used in this
form.

The points regarding position to be especially noted are these:—The patient should
be induced to carry the right arm with the
elbow a little in front of the body. A convenient and not an inelegant posture is insured
by placing the hand on the left side at the
waist. The left elbow and shoulder should be
habitually thrown rather back. In sleeping,
the patient should be encouraged, whatever
posture the body may assume, to keep the
right hand on the left shoulder or left side of
the neck. The left arm, if the posture be not
uneasy, should lie behind the body. The
woodcut upon p. 109 shows the action on
the spine of the sloping seat; and it is to
be observed that although this agent was

especially designed for lumbar curves, yet its
action does not stop at the loins, but affects
also the back, and is of great value in all
forms of dorsal curve; on this subject more
must be said in the future.

The exercises to be used in the weight-
bearing curve require very careful application, because there are certain points to be
considered which I have till now purposely
postponed. It is evident that if a weight
have produced upon its support a certain
effect, that consequence may arise from the
excess of weight (either in mass or in time),
or from the weakness of the support itself.
In practice both these forms of case present
themselves to our notice; and, besides, there
is a third variety: the support, originally
strong, has been injured, and the strength has
for the time disappeared. In each one of
these classes we must arrange differently our
mode of using exercises, and their intensity;
in the stronger and the rarer form, we may
employ them immediately after having by
the above-described devices produced some
effect upon the curves, and straightened them

to some extent. In the cases originally weak the work must be very gradually and lightly applied; in those **which have acquired de**bility, exercise—even the sloping **seat—must** be avoided until **a considerable improvement** in health has been obtained.

The exercises are chiefly directed to the left scapula. Firstly, after, by the other means described, a certain improvement has been effected, **and** if the amount of debility do not forbid, we may weight the left arm slightly. This may be done in any way; a piece of plumbers' **lead,** properly protected, squeezed **on above the** elbow, is a convenient plan. **Let the patient stand in the position of** a soldier at "attention," with the **right side** against the wall; **then slowly** lift the left hand and arm, at the same time throwing the head back; * or simply, **in the** same position, with the neck well bent back, let her only lift

---

* The throwing back of the head recommended in this and the following exercises, is prescribed in order to obviate action of the *trapezius* in lifting the shoulders, and to throw the whole burden of that movement on the *serratus magnus*.

the left shoulder several times. A stronger
exercise is to raise the left arm slowly from
the side until it forms a right angle with the
body, the head being well bent back. Again,
to swing the left arm strongly backwards and
forwards nearly at right angles to the body,
the hand pronated in front and supinated
behind; when the patient is strong enough, a
weight may be placed in the hand. The
influence on the ribs and spine of the two last
exercises will be much increased by the following device. A hook or staple on the patient's
left holds an accumulator attached to a handle
grasped by the patient on the right, with her
arm passing in front of her body, so that
the force draws the hand well over to the
left side.

If the weight-bearing curve be in the opposite direction, all these manœuvres must be
reversed; they are not to be used lightly nor
indiscriminately, and must be from time to
time rigidly watched.

The other form of dorsal deformity is far
more common, especially in the upper classes
of society, and when the surgeon has made so

accurate a diagnosis that he is sure of having
to do with a respiratory curve, he will be
aware that his treatment must be directed to
combating exaggerated pectoral breathing,
and the backward tendency of the right ribs.
However early, however advanced the case,
this must be one of his aims; indeed, if in the
earliest stages of the malady he could insure
these results, he would have done enough;
but the deformity usually comes under care in
a further advanced condition, and it is necessary, therefore, that he add means to obviate
lateral deviation and to restore normal position.

In the first place, it is very important that
the arrangement of dress should be conform-
able to health and functional activity. It is
the duty of the surgeon to examine carefully
into this point; nor should he rest satisfied
with a mere assurance that nothing tight is
worn. Let him rather not think it derogatory
to see the sort of corset which the patient
affects, particularly the hardness and resist-
ance of that part which overlies the abdomen;
let him, too, observe the amount of constriction
produced by petticoat-strings, also the weight

of the clothing. This is frequently considerable, especially in the colder months, when
breathing, being more rapid, should be less
constrained, but when the mere pressure by
gravity on the abdomen renders respiration
too pectoral. In cases where the curve is
rapidly increasing, part of this weight may be
suspended from the left shoulder, by means of
an arrangement something after the fashion
of braces. This can be managed without any
difficulty, and I have in some cases seen considerable improvement follow such change.

The positions to be enforced in this form of
curvature are aimed at two objects,—the retrocession of ribs and the lateral deviation. I
have, in speaking of weight-bearing curvature, described certain postures. They are
such as by bringing forward the base of the
right scapula, tend to prevent overaction of
that serratus on the ribs, and to increase the
vantage ground for such influence of the left
muscle—all attitudes which bring the right
elbow in front of the body, the left behind, are
desirable—the patient should be encouraged
to acquire as a habit, in walking and standing,

to keep the right hand on the left side of the
waist. In sitting, she may advantageously let
the arm cross still further, so that the hand
rests over the left thigh. In sleeping she
should lie on the right side, a small cushion
should be placed under the axilla, the right
arm, brought well forward, should be over the
left shoulder or left side of the neck, while the
left arm should if possible lie behind the body.
Let none, till he has tried them, consider these
matters trivial; the force at any given moment
of a single drop of water may be small, but
let one fall at every instant, and the aggregate
effect will soon be quite sufficiently marked.
Of the postures used to obviate the lateral
deviation the first and most important is again
the sloping seat. I would beg the reader to
refer back to p. 109, on which is the figure
representing the action of this device. It will
there be seen that though it was designed
originally for cases of lumbar curve, yet its
action does not stop at the loins, but is continued upward to the dorsal spine. When a
patient is placed upon the mechanical stool,
with the seat horizontal, and a plumb-line is

dropped along the back from the seventh
cervical vertebra, it will cross the spine once
at or near the ninth dorsal vertebra, the fourth
or fifth will be at a certain distance from the
line, and this distance may be measured by
callipers. If, then, the one end of the seat be
slowly and gradually raised to a certain
height, and this distance be again measured,
it will be found to have decreased in proportion to the amount of slope. In all but severe
cases we can by a considerable angle perfectly
straighten the dorsal spine; yet this is not
desirable, the exertion necessary to the posture
being too severe, and likely as in a case
related (p. 113) to produce evil results. We
must content ourselves with a less amount of
immediate effect, and in each case form our
judgment of the desirable angle from the
aggregate experience of its action in other
cases. The changes in the lumbar spine
must be called in counsel, and the diminution
in its rotation will prove useful as an index.
Before concluding all that I shall have to say
upon the value of this device, it may be well
to point out that its efficacy appears to me to

lie in the fact that it does not, like external
force, compel a passive spine into a certain
posture, but obliges the muscles themselves to
straighten out the abnormal curve, and accus-
toms them to keep the spine straight. Another
available but far less valuable posture is that
known as the lateral swing ; it is simply an
arrangement of a broad bandage into a loop,
comparable to a round towel suspended an
inch or two above a couch ; in this loop the
patient lies in such manner that the most
pronounced part of the curve lies on the
bandage, the rest of the figure reposing on
the couch on a lower level than the suspended
portion. If this device be properly managed,
it is advantageous to a certain extent ; but it
has many defects. It acts on a passive spine,
and therefore has no influence on the muscular
root of the deformity. The bandage, too, is
apt to slip, it therefore requires careful watching, and thus the patient cannot sleep in it,
which would otherwise be its most advantageous use.

The exercises, which are useful in this form
of curvature, are only those that influence the

respiratory movements of the chest and abdomen. All the experiments which I have
made show that such gymnastics (and many
are described by authors) as affect the spinal
muscles proper are futile. A point omitted
for clearness' sake from the etiological history
of the malady must, however, here be noticed.
If the surgeon watch the respiratory movements, either by touch or sight, as may be most
facile, he will, in all cases of increasing curvature, find that the abdomen is perfectly motionless—even during forced breathing—in the
deep breaths which he may require the patient
to take, this part of the body is singularly immobile. Let him go further, and direct the
patient to move the abdominal walls in and out,
and he will in a large proportion of cases find
that there is great difficulty in obeying his
instructions. The physicians and other medical
men to whom, as opportunity offered, I have,
in hospital and in my consulting-room, pointed
out this peculiarity, have been much struck
with the phenomenon : its correction is one
of the important objects in the physiological
treatment of this malady. In all cases marked

by much of such immobility, any attempt to teach at once the normal, alternating action of abdominal breathing is useless ; the patient must first be directed simply to draw in and throw outward the abdominal walls at any regular or irregular interval, and after a time these movements may be combined with those of the chest and diaphragm until a more normal form of breathing is acquired.

Other exercises are thus planned :—we desire to place the trunk with appendages in such posture that in respiration the right serratus shall be in a disadvantageous position, the left in the best possible position for acting with power on the ribs. And here it may be permitted me to call attention to a peculiarity of the methods which I advocate, for therein will be found to be their value. In order to keep the body upright, the erector-muscles of the spine must be called into action ; but if they act upon a spine which is rotated so that they lie, not at the middle but at one side, they must of necessity bend that spine to the other side. Hence to attack these muscles as the cause of crookedness, is like blaming water for flowing down the side of a hill; hence also that desuetude into which nearly all devices of orthopædy have fallen, and the sort of despair expressed concerning the action of those that still survive (p. 91). But if, on the other hand, we direct our attention to the torsion, and overcome that defect, then the erectors will not in contracting make the spine crooked. For this purpose, we, among other exercises, enforce certain actions of the serratus (the dorsal rotating muscle), in such wise that respiration shall affect the left ribs as much, the right as little as possible. If the patient be sufficiently strong we shall gain two objects at once, by letting her perform the exercise while seated on the sloping seat, thus. To the wall on each side of her sloping chair let hooks be fixed, and let these bear strong elastic cords terminating in handles, which she is to use in the following manner : the right arm is to cross in front of the body and hold the handle attached to the wall on the left, while the left hand passes behind the trunk and grasps the handle from the right. The amount of tension must be carefully regulated, so that it shall not be irksome, and yet shall draw the right scapula far forwards, and the left well back.

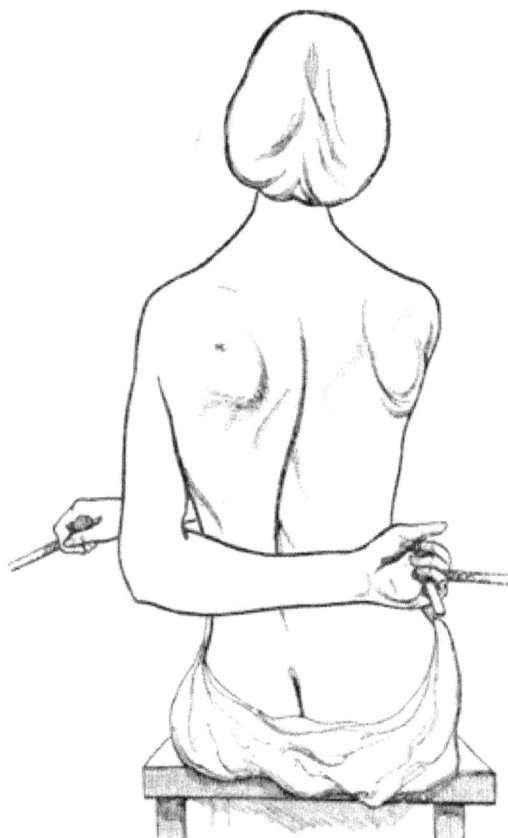

Left Respiratory Exercise.

The accompanying figure, from a photograph of a patient nearly cured, shows the kind of posture produced. Now the patient is to be directed to make several very deep

L

inspirations: let them be long and slow—if possible, only six to the minute ; the inspiration occupying more time than the expiration. By the different postures of the shoulder-blades the left serratus has more power than the right, and at each breath the left ribs will be chiefly used, giving a twist to the vertebræ contrary to the abnormal torsion ; but if the bodily powers be feeble, one exercise—either the sloping seat or the elastic cords—will be enough at a time.

Let the patient, while sitting on the sloping seat, keep the right arm crossed well over the chest ; then, taking a deep inspiration, throw back the left arm so that the hand describes part of a horizontal circle ; let this be repeated three times before taking a fresh breath and re-commencing the manœuvre. After a time some weight may advantageously be placed in the left hand.

These exercises, combined with the positions at repose, and the gradually increased use of the sloping seat, will suffice for the purposes indicated ; but, besides these, it is, in all but incipient cases, desirable to uphold the spine,

and to prevent retrocession of the right ribs
by the oblique bandage. The principles upon
which the device is founded have been already
explained; it will be only necessary to repeat
here that the forces are applied as nearly as
possible in directions transverse to the chords
of curves.

The fixed point is gained at the side of the
pelvis by means of a trapezoid piece of coutil,
which is held in place by a circular strap
passing around the upper part of the thigh.
From this pad runs, both in front and at the
back, a webbing strap to another pad placed
on the right over the most retrograde ribs;
and from this again, over both chest and back,
other straps pass to the left shoulder. The
straps are rendered elastic by intercalated
rings of india-rubber, and are, of course, provided with means of regulating tension. To
insure clearness of illustration, the bandage
has been depicted as though it were next the
skin; but it is not thus used, a very simple
arrangement of dress enabling the patient
to wear it outside the chemise and under-
clothing.

One of the objects fulfilled by this apparatus—namely, lateral action on the curves of

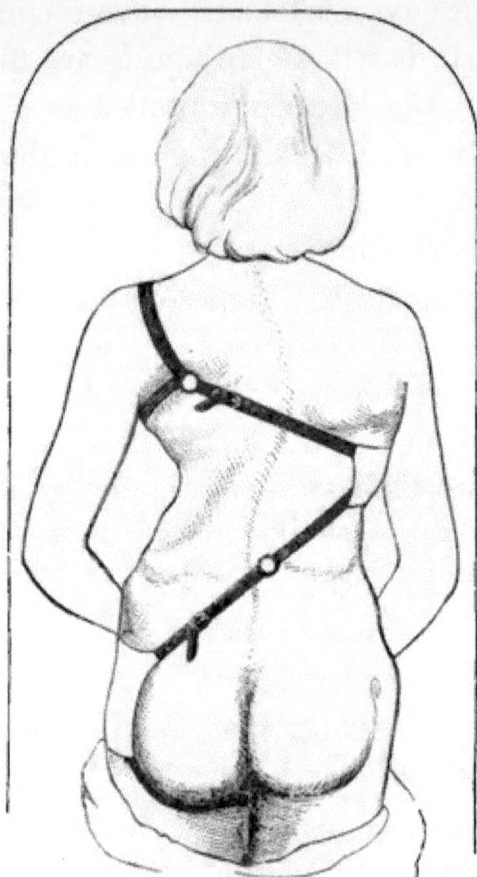

The Oblique Bandage.

(The pad on the right is a little too much at the side.)

the spine—has been discussed. The other—namely, such forward impulse to the right ribs as shall prevent, or aid in the cure of, rotation—is procured by difference of strength in the elastic rings before and behind, by certain checks to the elasticity of the latter, and by difference of tension regulated by the surgeon. This, with a little practice, is very easily achieved, care being taken to fix at a certain amount the difference of pressure. There are, however, some cases, chiefly those of old standing and much deformity, which require a somewhat modified bandage. Such changes are easily imagined, but I shall, when speaking of aggravated curvature, describe a form of band, devised on a rather different model.*

A certain custom or experience in the use of these different expedients will lead to a method that shall in each case develop their greatest value, and perhaps a few hints on the varying constitutions of patients affected with curvature will not be misplaced. Among

---

* The shoulder-sling is, in cases of weight-bearing curve, to be combined with this bandage simply by letting the point of the V-shaped strut be supported by the pad on the right side.

persons thus suffering we find all different forms of growth and constitution. The overgrown, pale, and slim young girl, whose form is popularly considered as the type and *beau ideal* for such distortion, is hardly, if at all, a more frequent victim than the strong, ruddy, and firmly built. But as the physical condition in these individuals is different, so will it be wise to make such variations in the method and time of our appliances as shall suit the particular case. The former sort will require at first only a small allowance of the exercises prescribed; the performance must be somewhat carefully watched. The use of the sloping seat also must be guarded. The same angle will affect a long spine more than a short one; but more especially it will be well to remember that weak muscles must not be over-exerted. On the other hand, the use of the bandage must at first, in the weaker spines, be more decided; and the lower pair of straps, more especially, must be made to do their work. Again, in such variety of constitutions, we shall, of course, find that medicinal treatment must vary. Some practitioners,

under the idea that all lateral distortion is a
result of debility, give quinine or iron in
every case; others, clinging to the notion that
some disease of bone produces the disease,
administer lime with the steel whenever a
lateral curve makes its appearance. In practice, however, we find that among a number
of people laterally distorted there shall be
all varieties of general condition—robustness,
anæmia, and, in fact, the only point of physical
resemblance shall be the curve itself; hence,
in many cases, medicine is quite unnecessary,
and had better therefore be omitted; in other
cases the general disturbance speaks for itself,
and must be treated. The curve itself and its
immediate cause are not to be benefited by
medicines; but when the severity of the distortion has produced loss of health—a not
uncommon circumstance—we shall find certain
tonics—quinine, iron, perhaps cod-liver oil,
and frequently iodine available;—that is to say,
they will be of some use; but these may be
administered to profusion, yet the pain and
the lassitude will continue until the local treatment has improved the condition of the back,

and then such symptoms will decrease. Concerning the choice of the above medicines, little need be said. The function of menstruation is not unfrequently greatly troubled in lateral curvature ; and very little experience of these cases leads one to observe, that this occurs more especially in the lumbar form of the malady. Such state will give a clue to the sort of medicinal treatment needed. Excessive languor, inedia, a shortness of breath, or a hacking cough, furnishes sufficient data for treatment in other cases ; while the absence of any such symptoms will warn us to withhold medicines where they are not wanted.

Perhaps it will be remembered that a promise has been made to show how the rotation-measure, whereof I have once or twice spoken, may be used as a means of determining whether a case is improving, or the reverse. If a patient with a dorsal curvature to the right present herself for treatment, it will be found, when she is subjected to test by this instrument, that the body will turn less to the right than to the left, and the difference will be commensurate with the

severity of the curves;* hence it follows that
if the patient get better the variation will
decrease, and *vice versâ*. Of course I do not
subject all patients presenting themselves for
treatment to this test—many circumstances,
besides the value of my time, would preclude
such practice; nevertheless I have, in a
goodly number of cases, kept a regular record
of these measurements, and subjoin one or
two such diaries:—

Miss C. B., aged nineteen, 1866.

	RIGHT.		LEFT.
19th February	30 deg.	40 deg.
25th April	26 „	36 „
10th June	30 „	35 „
15th August	36 „	35 „

Miss L. L., aged sixteen, 1866—1867.

	RIGHT.		LEFT.
27th July	40 deg.	70 deg.
24th August	35 „	61 „
21st September ..	40 „	60 „
19th October	50 „	59 „
16th November ..	54 „	58 „
14th January	58 „	58 „
11th February	60 „	58 „

* Very severe curves are, however, rather irregular
in their indications, and backs which have been kept
in steel supports have been thereby artificially stiffened;
their performance can not therefore be relied on.

Miss S. C., aged seventeen, 1867.

6th April				RIGHT.			LEFT.
6th April ..	..	..	25 deg.		..	..	40 deg.
,,	..	..	..	29 ,,	..	..	39 ,,
,,	..	..	..	32 ,,	..	..	38 ,,
,,	..	..	..	34 ,,	..	..	36 ,,
,,	..	..	..	38 ,,	..	..	37 ,,

A different way of measuring,—that by a silk thread stretched between the middle of the sacrum and the vertebra prominens,—may be adopted. There is, however, some difficulty in rendering such measurement very accurate, since the breadth of the spinous process is sufficient to give large margin for error, by carefully marking on the skin with ink, the inner and outer boundary of the bony prominence, and taking the centre as the point for measure; we can, however, obtain considerable exactitude in estimating lateral deviation in tolerably severe cases; but when the curvature is either slight in its commencement, or has advanced considerably towards cure, this is of very little avail. For instance :—

E. F., aged 22, came to me 15th November, 1865, with marked respiratory curvature to the right. She was a tall, rather slim girl; had of late lost health rapidly, and got thinner; appetite bad; complains of a good deal of dull pain at and about the right shoulder-blade and arm-pit, and also about the upper part of left ilium. There is evidently something vague and un-settled about this pain, as she finds difficulty in fixing its exact locality: it decreases when she has been for some time recumbent. Measurement of the curve gave—

		5th Dorsal $1\frac{7}{10}$ to right.		2nd Lumbar $1\frac{2}{10}$ to left.		
14th Dec., 1866.	,,	$1\frac{1}{10}$	,,	,,	$\frac{8}{10}$	,,
11th Feb.	,,	$\frac{9}{10}$	,,	,,	$\frac{7}{10}$	,,
1st March	,,	$\frac{5}{10}$	,,	,,	$\frac{4}{10}$	,,
25th April	,,	$\frac{2}{10}$	,,	,,	$\frac{2}{10}$	,,

August 15th.—There is still a perceptible, but scarcely (on the living body) a measurable distance; the line touches all the spinous processes, but does not lie over the centre of some of them.

September 27th, 1866.—The back is now perfectly straight; neither by eye nor manipulation, by measurement or the rotation test, can I find any difference.

Miss R——, aged $17\frac{1}{2}$ years was sent to me by my friend Dr. Cotton, October 12th, 1867, on account of the following conditions. During the last three or four months she having lost health, flesh, colour, and appetite, was taken to see Dr. Cotton, who found no signs of tubercle in the lung, but simply failure of vital power, he also saw upon her one of the usual steel supports that had been ordered her by one of that persuasion, and made by a practised maker. On questioning her the physician found that five months ago some apprehension had been excited by tendency to stoop, and she was taken to Mr. ——, who, ordering the usual mechanism, had seen her frequently, to screw up the levers in the interval.

In my presence the scaffolding was removed, and I found a dorsal curvature to the right pretty strongly marked; with those particular additions which I have always observed on backs that have for a length of time been supported by a stiff instrument—namely, that on first removal the spine remains in the same attitude, with a certain rigidity; and rotation is more marked than the lateral bend. After a time, and generally of a sudden, the back gives way and sinks into very considerable curves, and then the spine becomes again more flexible. There is considerable tenderness of the spinal muscles.

The patient is suffering under a morbid irritability; she flushes very easily, and has fainted once or twice on very slight occasions. I therefore ordered no exertion from position or exercise, but simply that she should remain erect but very little at a time, until a less exacting mode of support could be made.

25th.—The bandage was applied on the 18th, and she has since sat up more, and walked about a little, she is better generally; irritability is much less; the pain and tenderness of the spinal muscles have disappeared, or nearly so.

20th November.—The back has improved each time that I have seen it (about every ten or twelve days) and now the condition is very much better; her morbid irritability is gone, and although closely watching, I have seen none of that transient flush. The tenderness of the spinal muscles has also quite disappeared. The sloping seat, rising $1\frac{1}{2}$ inch to the foot, is ordered for her, which she is to use ten minutes twice in the day.

December 18th.—Still improving.

January 23rd, 1868.—During the last few weeks this young lady's improvement has been very rapid. There is now but very little lateral deviation; the rotation, however, is to a skilled examination very evident.

March 2nd.—This case is to be considered well. The patient's back is perfectly straight; she has gained health and flesh, her spirits are good, and she can take a fair amount of exercise.

April 17th.--I saw this patient again; the back remains perfectly straight.

CHAPTER IX.

ON SEVERE AND ON SLIGHT CURVATURE.

ALTHOUGH in the foregoing chapters the promise of our title "The Causes and Treatment of Lateral Curvature" has been realised, a few words may yet be advantageously employed in some considerations on the above subjects ; for, in order to preserve a certain clearness and succinctness of narrative, facts and illustrations have been taken from the typical condition—the state of medium severity —therefore the two extremes have been left nearly unnoticed.

Cases of very severe, or as we may call it, of exaggerated curvature, belong to the class of dorsal, and, I believe, always of the respiratory curves. I have never seen a case of lumbar curvature, nor of weight-bearing curve, approaching the degree of severity which I intend to designate by the term "exaggerated curve," a degree in which not any portion of the spine, but the angles of the right ribs, rotated far back form the hump. Such distortion may, and generally does, occur in the ordinary manner, commencing slowly and insidiously, either not treated at all, or not benefited by the treatment adopted, but going on gradually and steadily increasing; or it may arise in a much more sudden manner from internal disease. Some description has been given of the different shapes and positions of curvature produced by various lung-diseases (p. 74), the short high curvature of consumption, the longer and low curve of pneumonia, &c.; but if the whole lung, or pleural cavity, be affected, then we find a condition which, as far as the spinal distortion goes, precisely corresponds to the usual curvature.* There is the same relative amount of rotation and lateral flexion,—in fact, the same posture arising from identical muscular causes.

---

* That is, if the lung-mischief have been to the left; if the right lung have been affected, this difference of side must be superadded.

A number of these cases have come under my notice, and if the local disease improve, it is frequently very interesting to observe, how surely the curve keeps pace with its amendment. If, however, the respiratory malady does not improve, then the spinal distortion will, like its cause, remain stationary or get worse. The degree, to which, if the lung be seriously involved, the curvature may attain, depends upon the age at which the original disease has attacked the patient. Some of the worst distortions of the spine that I have ever seen have been produced by some severe mischief, rendering a lung useless, or all but useless, at a very early age. We, then, not only find distortion from unilateral respiration, but also from want of development of the ribs on one side. I have at the present time under my care a patient, aged 22, who is suffering under exaggerated curvature arising from pleuropneumia and empyema, which occurred when she was seven years of age. An old scar on the left side shows where the pus was evacuated. The whole of the left lung is carnefied, her lips and conjunctivæ are dusky from insufficient respiration, and the left side of the chest is so small that there hardly seems room for the heart. The upper ribs appear absent, so small are they, and the finger pressed under the clavicle comes against the venter of the scapula. The excessive crookedness and extreme rotation of the spine, cause the angle of the right ribs to form a prominent hump, visible even through a loose cloak.

Such very severe cases are exceptional: nevertheless, we not unfrequently meet with exaggerated distortion dependent either on the usual causes or from internal disease, and although either class cannot be considered curable, a good deal may be done to alleviate the suffering induced. The patients thus affected are generally incapable of any exertion, of standing or of sitting upright beyond a few minutes, and they are subject to certain severe pains on the left (the concave) side, about the lower intercostal spaces and upper parts of the abdomen : these pains also sometimes extend lower. Their origin is somewhat obscure : the peculiar position affecting muscular conditions may have something to do with them, or again

M

they may result from narrowing of the intervertebral foramina.

Our object in such cases can be simply to render life less painful and burdensome; we cannot—especially if the curve result from internal origin—hold out much prospect of producing any great alteration in form. The patient should as much as possible avoid sitting with the back unsupported, and her chair should be prominent at the region of the loins, so that the whole of the figure, not merely the shoulders, are upheld; and I certainly have always found benefit from making this seat slope from left to right—benefit, that is to say, in diminishing pain. Some sort of support is also necessary, but not such a one as renders, or endeavours to render, the figure immoveable; these are, after a certain time, very frequently discarded. In many cases, and those not among the most severe, the oblique bandage (p. 148) gives all necessary support, and patients have expressed themselves greatly relieved by its adoption, but other cases of a severer form, or suffering more pain from an equal amount of distortion, find advantage rather from a band, which gives more support over a larger surface, and which from its construction I have ventured to name "The Spiral Bandage."

The annexed plate will aid the comprehen-

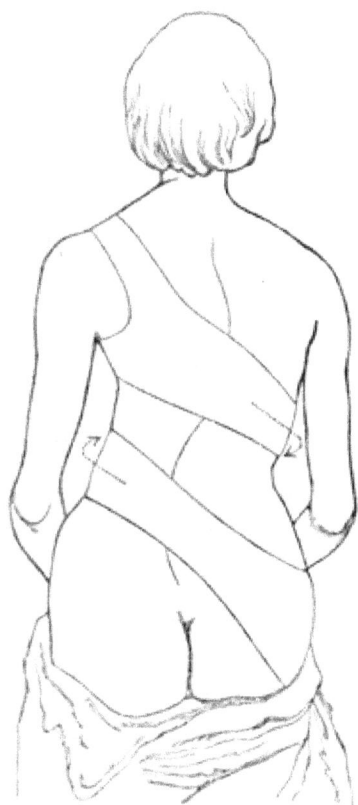

The Spiral Bandage.

sion of its action. A broad, irregularly trapezoid piece of coutil is secured on the upper

M 2

part of the right thigh by a round strap (if
this piece be properly shaped to the hip, it
has no tendency to slip), and is continued
round from the right hip to the left loin, where
it overlies the most prominent part of the
lumbar (secondary) curve; and then getting
narrower as it passes further round, it terminates in a strong india-rubber ring over
the cartilages of the false ribs.   On the left
shoulder another piece of coutil is secured by a
loop of the same material carefully fitted to the
part; from this loop the bandage passes round
the right side over the most pronounced dorsal
deviation, and tapering onward terminates
also in a strong india-rubber ring opposite to,
but a little higher than the one previously
named.   It now only remains to connect these
two rings by suitable broad straps, with means
of securing proper tension.   It is plain, from
this description, that when the india-rubber
rings are put upon the stretch, we have forces
at the most protuberant part of the back and
loins acting from the outer sides towards the
mesial line of the figure, tending therefore to
draw these parts into the straight position.

But this is not all. The direction of the
different parts of the bandage is such that the
force acts *round* the prominences—acts indeed
against rotation, and this power may be
increased by placing a pad on the eminences
under the bandage; or, as this beneath the
clothing increases the appearance of distortion, by making a gather or plait at that part.
The direction of the lateral and circular force
is marked in the woodcut by dotted lines and
arrow-heads. A few minor points, in details
of arrangement, may constitute just that difference, which will render such an apparatus
extremely comfortable or the reverse. For
instance, a cushion in front, where the rings
and connecting strap are situated, may be
made of a thin leather or of padded silk. The
loop at the arm causes in most patients no
inconvenience, in others it produces un-
comfortable pressure. In such case the discomfort may be entirely prevented by connecting the front part, where it glides under
the pectoralis, with one of the india-rubber
rings by means of a piece of elastic webbing.

This bandage I have found to be extremely

advantageous in relieving the pain, the liability to fatigue, the impossibility of sitting or standing upright for any length of time, and the sense of prostration such sufferers experience when obliged to go through a little more exertion than usual. Several such patients are now under my care, and although I do not intend to give cases of this far advanced distortion, a few remarks on one or two of them may be to the point:—

One lady, aged 38, has devoted nearly all the early part of her life to instruments, gymnastics, couches, &c. In 1855 she was still wearing a spinal support, sometimes during both night and day. The instrument was very fatiguing, and its wear injured her health greatly. She went to the sea-side, and remained recumbent for nearly two years; then had a lighter instrument, but found the pain continue, and her health again began to give way. During the last few years she has worn no appliance, as she says that she feels more comfortable without them. She came to me at the end of 1867, being only capable of sitting up for a few minutes, and then with

pain. Having caused a chair to be arranged
after the principles given above, I then had a
spiral bandage constructed. Since that time
she has been able to go about a good deal
more without nearly so much fatigue, and in
the early part of this present May she sat out
a whole oratorio without feeling over-tired.

Another lady, aged 28, came to me in
June, 1866, with a strong curvature, and a
severe support, in consequence of which she
was suffering very considerable pain. As
soon as a spiral bandage could be constructed,
I let her change the one appliance for the
other. Formerly, in taking a railway journey,
she was obliged to have two seats, with a
board, india-rubber cushions, &c., and travel
horizontally, and even then suffered much.
At Christmas time last year she, by tighten-
ing the spiral bandage a little, was able to
travel sitting upright for nearly two hundred
miles with but very little discomfort.

The few words which I would say on the
subject of very slight curvatures rather relate
to diagnosis than to treatment. The natural

anxiety of a mother that her daughter should
grow up straight, leads many parents to take
a girl to someone reputed skilled in this
class of case; in order either that any desirable treatment might be adopted, or that her
parental fears may be set at rest. Under
such circumstances it is, of course, necessary
that a correct judgment should be formed and
given. In such cases the probability is that
some unevenness of the two shoulders will
have caused the lady's doubts, and it is upon
the sort of difference in height of those parts
that I would speak; for the right or the left
shoulder may assume an habitual attitude a
little higher than the other, and yet there
may be no spinal deviation.

The scapula is very moveable; it may be
temporarily lifted by the action of the trapezius and serratus to a considerable height, or
it may, through some awkward trick of habit,
be kept permanently above the level of the
opposite side by similar muscular action; but
in all these postures the dorsum of the bone
will not alter its aspect; like its fellow of the
opposite side, it looks backwards and a little

outwards, and but very little or not at all
upwards. If the acromion be brought forward,
the dorsum of the one bone will look more
outward than that of the other. But something more than this happens when the
shoulder is displaced by deeper causes. At
p. 64 is given an account of the manner in
which the scapula is pushed back from beneath
by the retrocession of the ribs. The bone
overlies the upper ribs from the second to the
seventh; its lower angle just touching the one
last enumerated, when the arms hang by the
side. Now we know that the fifth dorsal
vertebra is that which has most deviated, and
the fifth rib the one that in its lever-like action
recedes most. Hence it is the lower part of
the scapula which is most pushed back, the
upper costa being but very little, if at all,
affected. The bone then becomes too horizontal, the dorsum will look too much *upwards*,
and the lower angle will protrude too far
back—stick out too much. This is the position which should inspire anxiety; the mere
elevation of the shoulder has nothing to do
with spinal curve. Even this too horizontal

position alone is not to satisfy the surgeon
that curvature exists. He must also examine
the relative position of ribs on both sides of
the back, must ascertain if rotation have taken
place (p. 60) ; that is to say, if the peculiar
position of the scapula be produced by its
being pressed backward by the ribs themselves. I have been induced to insist with a
certain minuteness on these points, because, in
several instances, medical men bringing me
patients have been somewhat inclined to doubt
my assurance that no lateral curve existed,
referring again after such negation to the
heightened shoulder ; but all those friends have
acknowledged to me that subsequent events
have proved the correctness of my diagnosis.

Again, it has appeared well to lay such
stress upon this subject, because it is closely
connected with what may be called " hysterical spine." There is, in my experience,
no mock disease so common as an hysterical simulation of dorsal malady. But in
nearly every such case diagnosis is not difficult. The pain or flinching upon slight contact, the ease with which steady pressure is

borne, either absence of any rotation and curve, or presence of one simple curve, which increases while the patient knows herself watched, and disappears nearly or entirely when her attention is directed elsewhere, with other signs, are all very strongly marked, and afford a sufficient ground for undoubting diagnosis. Sometimes, however, we meet with mixed cases,—cases in which there is weakness of the spine, with slight rotation, a tendency to, rather than actual distortion, and mingled therewith a highly hysterical condition,—such a case was quite lately sent me by Dr. Theodore Davis of Clevedon ; others also presenting extreme difficulty of diagnosis and of treatment, have come to my notice. They are, nevertheless, unusual. The points, however, regarding the position of the shoulder and the occurrence of hysterical complication must be well known to the surgeon examining these cases ; lest he fall into the error, sometimes committed, of subjecting to long treatment a spine which is perfectly healthy.

INDEX.

A.

		Page
ABDOMEN, compression of	.. ..	35, 95
„ immobility of in **dorsal curve**	.. ..	143
„ muscles of, producing **secondary curve**	.. ..	45
Amputated arm, curvature from	.. ..	38
Awkward habits, influence of	.. ..	53
Axis of rotation	.. ..	21

B.

BANDAGE, lumbar	.. ..	.. 119
„ oblique	.. ..	.. 149
„ spiral	.. ..	.. 162

C.

CASES of dorsal curvature	.. ..	.. 153
„ lumbar curvature	.. ..	.. 121
Case-taking by rotation measure	.. ..	.. 153
„ „ string measure	.. :. ..	.. 154
Causation of curvature reconsidered	.. ..	37
Cause, position as	.. ..	75
Causes of dorsal curvature	.. ..	26
„ normal curves	.. ..	7
Changes in spine, consecutive	.. .. ..	83
„ of form, anterior	.. ..	67
Characteristics of curvature	.. ..	3

Page

Classification of treatment 99
Compression of intervertebral substance 84
Constitutions, manifold 150
Consumptive curve 36
Cruveilhier, measurements by 85
Curability, signs of 81

D.

DEBILITY of spinal muscles 3
Definitions 27
Degeneration, muscular 82
Diary of rotation 153
Diagnosis of different curvatures .. 59
          „   slight curvature 167
Differential diagnosis 61
Directness of treatment 104
Divisions of treatment 99
Dorsal curve, treatment of 129
Dress, management of 137

E.

ELASTICITY of ligaments 88
      „   „ spine 12
Exaggerated curvature 158
      „   „   examples of 161
Exercise for lumbar curve 115
Exercises for respiratory curve 141
      „   weight-bearing curve 135

F.

FORMATION of spine 5
Flexibility, lateral, of spine .. 16

H.

Page

HABITS, awkward, influence of 53
Head upheld by shoulder 8
High light, examine by 60
Hip, projection of 63
Horizontal posture of scapula 169
Hysteric curve 170

I.

INFANTILE spine 6
Internal causes, curves from 74, 159
Intervertebral substance in curvatures 86
,, ,, disease of 4

L.

LAMENESS, influence of.. 51
Lateral flexibility of spine 16
Lever-like action of ribs 32
Ligaments, elasticity of 87
,, normal action of 12
Light, advantages of high 60
Limb movement, influence of 18
Lumbar bandage 119
,, curve, primary causes of 48
,, ,, secondary causes of 42
,, ,, treatment of causes of .. 106
Lumbar muscles, diagram of 55
,, produce lumbar rotation .. 54
Lung-disease, its curves .. 36

M.

MEASUREMENT of curves by rotation .. 153
,, ,, cord .. 154

Page

Measurement of normal curves 9
Medicinal treatment 151
Medico-Chirurgical Society, expressions at .. 98
Movement, limb, influence of 18
    ,, normal, of vertebræ 6
    ,, undulatory, of spine 49
Multiple curves 28
Muscular degenerations 82
Myatomy, spinal, history of.. 57

N.

Normal curves, cause of 7
    ,,   ,, measure of 9
    ,, rotation, measure of 15
    ,,   ,, production of 30

O.

Oblique bandage 147
Opinions, orthopædic 97
Orthopædic support 93

P.

Pain in severe curvature 161
Paralysis of respiratory muscles.. 3
    ,, spinal muscles 3
Pectoral breathing in dorsal curvature .. 35
Peculiarities of lateral curve 2
Pelvis, backward projection of, in lumbar curve .. 62
    ,, infantile posture of 6
    ,, lateral projection, late symptom 62
Plan of treatment 99
Pleuritic curvature 37, 159
Pneumonic curvature.. .. .. 37, 159

Page

Position as cause of curvature 75
 ,, remedial of dorsal curve 138
 ,,   ,,   lumbar curve.. 108
 ,,   ,,   weight-bearing curve 133
Primary and secondary curves 27
Principles of treatment 90
Projection of hip 62
 ,, ,, ribs 64
 ,, ,, scapula 64, 169
Prone position, influence of.. 101

R.

Raphé of back 66
Recumbency, influence of 89, 101
Resiliency of spine.. 13
Respiration, male and female 34
Respiratory action of serratus 34
 ,, curve, diagnosis of 69
 ,, exercise 145
Ribs, levers in rotation 32
 ,, projection backwards of 64
Right arm, over-action of 4
Rotation, dorsal, produced by 33
 ,, lumbar, produced by 54
 ,, measurement of 16
 ,, measurer in diagnosis.. 69
 ,, normal, produced by 14

S.

Scapula, diagnostic posture of 168
 ,, projection of 64
Secondary and primary curves 27
 ,, lumbar curve 42
Section of spinal muscles 55

Page

Serratus magnus, exercise of 145

,, ,, respiratory action of 34

,, ,, rotating power of 30

,, ,, supports weight of arm.. 33

Severe curves.. 158

Shape of vertebræ 11

Shoe, high, for lumbar curves 114

Shoulder-sling 131

Signs of curability.. 81

Slight curvature 167

Sloping seat, dorsal curve 139

,, ,, lumbar curve.. 109

Spastic contraction 3

Spiral bandage 162

Sternum, deviation of 67

Stool, mechanical 110

Straight infantile spine 6

Supports, orthopædic 40, 93

Supports transverse to curve 102

T.

Tension of ligaments 84

Theories, review of 3

Traction, longitudinal, effects of.. 91

Transverse processes in lumbar curve 56

Treatment, medicinal 151

,, principles of 90

U.

UMBILICUS, displacement of.. 67

Undulatory movements of spine.. .. 49

Uneven distribution of weight 51

V.

VERTEBRÆ, disease of 4

,, position of.. 6

,, in curvature rarely changed 86

W.

Page

WEAKNESS in severe curves 161
   ,,   of spinal muscles 3
Weight-bearing curve diagnosis 71
   ,,   ,, curvature from 38
   ,,   ,,   ,, treatment of .. 130
Weight-carrying, influence of 19
Weight of heart as cause 4
   ,, ,, liver as cause 4
   ,, uneven distribution of 4

X.

Xiphoid cartilage, deviation of .. 67

LONDON: PRINTED BY W. CLOWES AND SONS, DUKE STREET, STAMFORD STREET,
AND CHARING CROSS.